Economics of Public and Private Healthcare and Health Insurance in India

This book critically examines the public and private health care systems in India. Analysing the current scenario of health insurance in India, it studies the inadequacy of public health care services and unaffordability of private health care facilities. The volume investigates government-sponsored health insurance schemes and advocates for universal health insurance coverage. It details India's per capita health expenditure and provides policy inputs on how health care systems and insurance coverage can be improved in the country. Further, it explores the financial parameters of health insurers and stand-alone private health insurance companies and discusses the adverse impact of the COVID-19 pandemic on Indian health care.

An insightful read on the state of health care in India, this book will be of interest to researchers and academics working in the fields of insurance, health care administration and management, public health policy and practice, health and social care, medical sociology, and sociology and social policy. It will also be useful for think tanks and policymakers.

Brijesh C. Purohit is Professor at Madras School of Economics (MSE), Chennai, India. Prior to joining the MSE in 2008, he served at various academic institutions in India which include the Administrative Staff College of India, Hyderabad; Institute of Development Studies, Jaipur; Indian Institute of Health Management and Research, Jaipur; National Institute of Public Finance and Policy, New Delhi; and Central University of Rajasthan. His career, spanning more than 30 years, includes research, teaching, training and consultancy. He was also South Asian Visiting Scholar at Queen Elizabeth College, Department of Development Studies, University of Oxford, UK. He holds a PhD in economics from the Institute for Social and Economic Change, Bangalore, India.

Economics of Public and Private Healthcare and Health Insurance in India

Second Edition

Brijesh C. Purohit

Routledge
Taylor & Francis Group

LONDON AND NEW YORK

Second edition published 2024
by Routledge
4 Park Square, Milton Park, Abingdon, Oxon, OX14 4RN

and by Routledge
605 Third Avenue, New York, NY 10158

Routledge is an imprint of the Taylor & Francis Group, an informa business

© 2024 Brijesh C. Purohit

First edition published by SAGE 2020

British Library Cataloguing-in-Publication Data
A catalogue record for this book is available from the British Library

ISBN: 978-1-032-51027-9 (hbk)
ISBN: 978-1-032-61565-3 (pbk)
ISBN: 978-1-032-61566-0 (ebk)

DOI: 10.4324/9781032615660

Typeset in Sabon
by Deanta Global Publishing Services, Chennai, India

Contents

List of Figures   *vi*
List of Tables   *viii*
Preface   *xiv*
Acknowledgements   *xv*

1 Introduction   1

2 All India Scenario of Health Facility Utilisation   5

3 Sustainable Development Goals and Health Insurance in
   India   60

4 Ayushman Bharat (MODI Care) and Other Government-
   Sponsored Health Insurance in India   107

5 Role of Public and Private Sectors in Health Insurance   127

6 Demand for Health Insurance in India   156

7 Conclusions and Policy Imperatives   189

8 Role of Health Insurance in Post-pandemic Time   193

Index   *199*

Figures

2.1   Current Health Expenditure in India and Other Southeast
Nations (in US$ Per Capita for the Years 2000, 2010 and 2016) 10

2.2   Current Health Expenditure in India and Other Southeast
Nations (as % of GDP for the years 2000, 2010 and 2016)   11

2.3   Government Health Expenditure (GHE) and out of Pocket
Health Expenditures (OOPE) as % of GDP (2015–16)   13

2.4   Government Health Expenditure (GHE) and Out of Pocket
Health Expenditures (OOPE) in Rs. Per capita (2015–2016)   13

2.5   Government Health Expenditure (GHE) by Central and
State Government and by Govt Insurance   14

2.6   Inpatient, Outpatient and Other Components in Health
Care Expenditure (2015–2016)   16

2.7   Health Care Expenditure across Primary, Secondary and
Tertiary Care in India (2015–2016)   17

2.8   Per Capita Availability of Sub-centres in BAIAS and AAIAS   20

2.9   Per Capita Availability of PHCs in BAIAS and AAIAS   20

2.10   Per Capita Availability of CHCs in BAIAS and AAIAS   21

2.11   Per Capita Availability of Subdivisional Hospitals in
BAIAS and AAIAS   21

2.12   Per Capita Availability of District Hospitals in BAIAS and
AAIAS   22

2.13   Per Capita Availability of Hospital Beds in BAIAS and AAIAS   27

2.14   Variation of Per Capita AYUSH Hospitals in AAIAS and BAIAS 30

2.15   Variation of Per Capita AYUSH Dispensaries in AAIAS
and BAIAS   30

2.16   AYUSH Doctors in BAIS and AAIAS   34

2.17   ANMs in BAIS and AAIAS   34

2.18   RN and RNMs in BAIS and AAIAS   35

2.19   LHVs in BAIS and AAIAS   35

2.20   Pharmacists in BAIS and AAIAS   36

2.21   Sources of treatment in India: A Synoptic View   49

2.22   Per Capita Health Expenditures on Health in BAIAS and AAIAS 50
2.23   Per Capita Government Health Expenditures in BAIAS and
        AAIAS   50
3.1   Expenditures among Three Broad Health Insurances in India   65
3.2   Polyclinics under CGHS in Major Cities (2018)   69
3.3   Empanelled Clinics and Diagnostic Centres under CGHS (2015) 73
3.4   Total Hospitals and Diagnostic Centres Empanelled under
        CGHS (2015)   73
3.5   Eye and Dental Clinics Empanelled under CGHS (2015)   74
3.6   Shortfall between targets and achievements in enrolment of
        RSBY in major states (2012–2017)   81
3.7   Hospitalisations by smart card holders of RSBY in 2012–13   87
5.1   Health Insurance Premium: Public, Private and Stand-alone
        companies (Rs. crore) (2010–2017)   131
5.2   Health Insurers' Net profits: Public, Private and
        Stand-alone companies (Rs. crore) (2010–2017)   132
5.3   Classification of Health Insurance Business   132
5.A4.1 Organisational Structure of BASIX Health Insurance   151
5.A4.2 Coverage and Experience in Different Phases of Karuna
        Trust Trends in Monthly Claims in Two Pilot Areas   154

Tables

1.A.1	Population norms for Health Infrastructure in Rural India (Public Health Care System)	4
1.A.2	Health Manpower Norms	4
2.1	Key Health Financing Indicators for India across NHA Rounds	12
2.2	Current Health Expenditures (2015–2016)	15
2.3	Rural Health Care Facilities in India across Major 20 States	18
2.4	Per Capita Availability of Rural Facilities across Indian States	19
2.5	Government Hospitals and Beds: Numbers: Rural, Urban and Per Capita Terms	23
2.6	Government Hospitals and Beds: Numbers: Rural, Urban and Per Capita Terms	24
2.7	Government Hospitals and Beds: Numbers: Rural, Urban and Per Capita Terms	25
2.8	Government Allopathic Doctors and Dental Surgeons Numbers and Per Capita Terms	26
2.9	Distribution of AYUSH Hospitals and Dispensaries across States and Systems	28
2.10	Per Capita Availability AYUSH Facilities AAIAS	29
2.11	Per Capita Availability AYUSH Facilities BAIAS	29
2.12	State/UT wise AYUSH Registered Practitioners (Doctors) in India as on January 1, 2017	31
2.13	State/UT wise Registered Nurses and Pharmacists in India as on January 1, 2017	32
2.14	State/UT wise PHC Doctors, Specialist at CHCs and Health Workers in India as on January 1, 2017	33
2.15	An Overview of Crude Prevalence of Mental Illness and Substance Abuse in India (2015–2016)	36
2.16	Prevalence of Different Mental Disorders	37
2.17	Principal Components Using 64 Variables	38
2.18	Regression result for Moderate Mental Disorder	38
2.19	Regression Result for High Mental Disorder	38

2.20	Regression Result for Screener Positive in Mental Disorder	39
2.21	Regression Result for Any Substance Use in Mental Disorder	39
2.22	Regression Result for Other Substance Use in Mental Disorder	40
2.23	Regression Result for Tobacco Use in Mental Disorder	40
2.24	Regression Result for Epilepsy in Mental Disorder	40
2.25	Regression Result for Suicidal Risk in Mental Disorder	40
2.26	Source of Treatment in India: Public and Private Shares	41
2.27	Source of Treatment in India: Public-private shares in Rural-Urban areas	42
2.28	Source of Treatment in Below All India Average Income States (BAIAS)	43
2.29	Source of Treatment in Rural Areas in Below All India Average Income States (BAIAS)	44
2.30	Source of Treatment in Urban Areas Below All India Average Income states (BAIAS)	45
2.31	Source of Treatment in Above All India Average Income States (AAIAS)	46
2.32	Source of Treatment in Rural Areas of Above All India Average Income States (AAIAS)	47
2.33	Source of Treatment in Urban Areas of Above All India Average Income States (AAIAS)	48
2.A1.1	Five-Year Plan Outlays: Pattern of Central Allocation (Total for the Country & Union MOHFW) (Rs. in crore)	51
2.A1.2	Current Health Expenditures (2015–2016) by Health care Functions	52
2.A1.3	Primary, Secondary and Tertiary Care Expenditures	53
2.A1.4	Per Capita Incomes (2015–2016)	54
2.A2.1	Major Correlations in PCA	55
2.A3.1	Key Indicators for NHA Above and Below All India Average States (2015–2016)	57
2.A3.2	Out of Pocket Expenditure (OOPE)	57
2.A3.3	Population, GDP and General Government Expenditure	57
2.A3.4	Total and Government Health Expenditures	58
2.A3.5	Out of Pocket Expenses for AAIAS	58
2.A3.6	Population, GDP and General Government Expenditure AAIAS	58
3.1	Current Status of Health Related SDG Targets – Indian Scenario	61
3.2	Total Health Care Expenditure and Out of Pocket Expenses in 2015–2016	62
3.3	Difference in Per cent GDP of THE and OOPE	63
3.4	Health Insurance Expenditure (2015–2016) under Different Schemes	66
3.5	Total, Per Capita Expenditure and No. of Beneficiaries in CGHS (2011–2018)	67

3.6	CGHS Dispensaries and Beneficiaries (2001–2018)	68
3.7	Distribution of AYUSH Dispensaries/Wellness Centres (2018)	70
3.8	Distribution of Cards and Beneficiaries under CGHS (2018)	71
3.9	Distribution of Doctors under CGHS in Major Cities (2018)	72
3.10	Coverage of ESIS (as on March 31, 2017)	76
3.11	Trends in Coverage, Income and Expenditure on ESIS	76
3.12	Income and Expenditure of Employees State Insurance Corporation (ESIC) in India (Growth 2001–2013)	77
3.13	State-wise Expenditure Incurred on Provision of Medical Care under Employees State Insurance Corporation (ESIC) in India (2009–2010)	78
3.14	State-wise Contributions under ESIS	79
3.15	Budget Allocation for RSBY (2007–2017)	82
3.16	Selected State-wise Hospitals Empanelment under RSBY (2016–2017)	84
3.17	Selected State-wise Number of Smart Cards Issued under Rashtriya Swasthya Bima Yojana (RSBY) in India (2008–2009 to 2012–2013 and 2016–2017)	85
3.18	Persons Hospitalised under Rashtriya Swasthya Bima Yojana (RSBY) in India (2008–2009 to 2012–2013 and 2016–2017)	86
3.19	State-wise Total number of beneficiaries under RSBY (2008–2014)	88
3.20	State-wise Total number of Workers of unorganised sector benefitted under RSBY (2013–14)	89
3.A.1	Status of CGHS as on 2000	90
3.A.2	City-wise CGHS Dispensaries	91
3.A.3	Empanelled Hospitals and Diagnostic Centre under CGHS	92
3.A.4	Brief Description of Benefits, Contributory Conditions, Duration of Benefits and the Scale of Benefits of ESIS	93
3.A.5	Income and Expenditure of Employees State Insurance Corporation (ESIC) in India (2001 to 2007, as on 31st March)	95
3.A.6	Selected State-wise Cash and Other Benefits under ESIS	97
3.A.7	Selected State-wise Other Benefits Given under ESIS	99
3.A.8	Families Enrolled under RSBY (2012–17, States and All India)	101
5.1	Varistha Mediclaim Policy	129
5.2	Rashtriya Swasthya Bima Policy	129
5.3	Parivar Mediclaim Policy	129
5.4	Vidyarthi Mediclaim Policy	130
5.5	Universal Health Insurance Scheme	130
5.6	Number of Persons Covered under Health Insurance (Excluding Pa & Travel Insurance Business)	133
5.7	Claims Ratios across Sectors	133

5.8	Claims Ratios across Types of Business	134
5.9	Per cent of NGOs in Health Sector	135
5.10	Coverage of Population and Inpatient/Outpatient Care (Pertaining to 16 Community Financed Health Insurance Schemes)	136
5.11	Inventory of Non-Governmental, Non-profit Health Insurers (Schemes Covering Inpatient Care Only) in India	137
5.12	Community Health Insurance in Three Districts of Uttar Pradesh	139
5.A1.1	Some of the Health Insurance Plans offered by Private Insurance Companies in India at a Glance	142
5.A1.2	Health Insurance Products Cleared during the Financial Year 2011–2012	144
5.A2.1	Gramin Swasthya Micro Insurance	144
5.A2.2	National Mediclaim Plus	144
5.A2.3	National Mediclaim Policy	145
5.A3.1	Health Insurance Premium: Public, Private and Stand-alone Companies (Rs. crore) (2010–2017)	145
5.A3.2	Health Insurers' Net Profits: Public, Private and Stand-alone Companies (Rs. crore) (2010–2017)	145
5.A3.3	Incurred Claims Ratio: Public-Sector Non-life Insurers	146
5.A3.4	Incurred Claims Ratio: Private Sector Non-life Insurers	147
5.A4.1	BASIX: Some Characteristics	149
5.A4.1a	BASIX: Some Additional Characteristics	149
5.A4.2	Grameen Arogya Raksha Component of BASIX	150
5.A4.3	Self-Health Group Parivaar Beema of BASIX	150
5.A4.4	Number of BASIX Health Insurance Clients by Gender as of November 30, 2006	151
5.A4.5	Performance in Claims Servicing as of December 26, 2006	151
5.A4.6	Coverage and Experience in Phases I and II	154
6.1	Overall Health Insurance Coverage in India (2015–2016)	157
6.2	Any Health Insurance	158
6.2(a)	Any Health Insurance (Marginal Effects)	158
6.3	RSBY	159
6.3(a)	RSBY (Marginal Effects)	159
6.4	State HIS	160
6.4(a)	State HIS (Marginal effects)	160
6.5	HITEMPloyer	160
6.5(a)	HITEMPloyer (Marginal Effects)	161
6.6	Private Health Insurance	161
6.6(a)	Private Health Insurance (Marginal Effects)	161
6.7	Private Health Insurance for Females	162
6.7(a)	Private Health Insurance for Females (Marginal Effects)	162

6.8	HITEMPloyer for Females	162
6.8(a)	HITEMPloyer for Females (Marginal Effects)	163
6.9	HI ABPL	163
6.9(a)	HI ABPL (Elasticities)	164
6.10	SHI	164
6.10(a)	SHI (Elasticities)	164
6.11	RSBY	165
6.11(a)	RSBY(Elasticities)	165
6.12	CHI	165
6.12(a)	CHI Elasticities	166
6.13	Private Insurance	166
6.13(a)	Private Insurance (Elasticities)	166
6.14	Private Insurance Females	167
6.14(a)	Private Insurance Females (Elasticities)	167
6.15	Any Health Insurance (Urban BPL)	168
6.15(a)	Any Health Insurance (Urban BPL) (Elasticities)	168
6.16	State Health Insurance (Urban BPL)	168
6.16(a)	State Health Insurance (Urban BPL)	169
6.17	RSBY (Urban BPL)	169
6.17(a)	RSBY (Urban BPL) (elasticities)	169
6.18	HITEMP(Urban BPL)	170
6.18(a)	HITEMP(Urban BPL) (Elasticities)	170
6.19	PrHI(Urban BPL)	170
6.19(a)	PrHI(Urban BPL) (Elasticities)	171
6.20	PrHI(Urban BPL) (Females)	171
6.20(a)	PrHI (Urban BPL) (Females) (Elasticities)	171
6.21	Any Health Insurance (Urban Above BPL)	172
6.21(a)	Any Health Insurance (Urban Above BPL) (Elasticities)	172
6.22	State Health Insurance (Urban Above BPL)	172
6.22(a)	State Health Insurance (Urban Above BPL) (Elasticities)	173
6.23	RSBY (Urban Above BPL)	173
6.23(a)	RSBY (Urban Above BPL) (Elasticities)	173
6.24	CHI (Urban Above BPL)	174
6.24(a)	CHI (Urban Above BPL) (Elasticities)	174
6.25	PrHI (Urban Above BPL)	174
6.25(a)	PrHI (Urban Above BPL) (Elasticities)	175
6.26	PrHI Females (Urban Above BPL)	175
6.26(a)	PrHI Females (Urban Above BPL)	175
6.27	SHI MP	176
6.27(a)	SHI MP	176
6.28	RSBY MP	177
6.28(a)	RSBY MP	177
6.29	PHI MP	177

6.29(a)	PHI	178
6.30	SHI MP ABPL Urban	178
6.30(a)	SHI MP ABPL Urban	178
6.31	RSBY MP ABPL Urban	179
6.31(a)	RSBY MP ABPL Urban	179
6.32	CHI MP ABPL Urban	179
6.32(a)	CHI MP ABPL Urban	180
6.33	PHI MP ABPL Urban	180
6.33(a)	PHI MP ABPL Urban	180
6.34	PHI ONLY FEMALES MP ABPL Urban	181
6.34(a)	PHI ONLY FEMALES MP ABPL Urban	181
6.35	SHI MP Rural BPL	181
6.35(a)	SHI MP Rural BPL	182
6.36	RSBY MP Rural BPL	182
6.36(a)	RSBY MP Rural BPL	182
6.37	CHI MP Rural BPL	183
6.37(a)	CHI MP Rural BPL	183
6.38	PHI MP Rural BPL	183
6.38(a)	PHI MP Rural BPL	184
6.39	PHI Females Only MP Rural BPL	184
6.39(a)	PHI Females Only MP Rural BPL	184
6.40	SHI Above BPL MP	185
6.40(a)	SHI Above BPL MP	185
6.41	RSBY Above BPL MP	185
6.41(a)	RSBY Above BPL MP	186
6.42	CHI Above BPL MP	186
6.42(a)	CHI Above BPL MP	186
6.43	PHI Above BPL MP	187
6.43(a)	PHI Above BPL MP	187
6.44	PHI Above BPL Females MP	187
6.44(a)	PHI Above BPL Females MP	188

Preface

Health care has been recognised the world over as an essential ingredient for human well-being. However, despite a good deal of policies and budgetary efforts, there seems to be a notable lacuna in the system. In India, despite a policy emphasis on Health for All, there remain significant gaps in the health care and health insurance systems. This book deals with analysing the Indian health care sector and role of health insurance, both in the public and private sectors in the country. It uses various data sources published by government organisations. It includes central and state budgets, Census of India, National Sample Survey (NSSO), statistical abstracts of different states and data from National Family Health Survey. The book compares and contrasts poorer and richer states.

Acknowledgements

This book is borne out of my interest in health economics and financing. I thank all journals and publishers that have provided inputs for the literature reviewed and analysed here.

I am grateful to my family members and friends for all the support to grow in my academic areas of interest. I am especially thankful to my late elder brother, Dr Mahesh C. Purohit, for encouraging me to carry out new academic work. I am also grateful to Routledge for bringing out the second edition of this book.

Chapter 1

Introduction

In India, state governments shoulder the major responsibility of providing health care. After independence, a model of health care delivery based on the Bhore Committee[1] recommendations was initially adopted. It provided a blueprint for the development of a three-tier system of health care delivery which comprised primary, secondary and tertiary levels of health care. Health care at these levels is provided by both public and private health care providers.

The primary level of health care consists of community health centres (CHCs), primary health centres (PHCs) and sub-centres (SCs). The sub-district hospitals come under the category of secondary health care and the tertiary level of health care includes the district hospitals and medical colleges. The system development is based on certain population norms. These are: in plain areas, every sub-centre covers a population of 5000 and in hilly or tribal areas it covers only a population of 3000. Likewise, a primary health centre covers a population 30,000 in plain areas against 20,000 of the population in hilly or tribal areas. CHCs in plain areas cover a population of 120,000, while in hilly areas this proportion of the population is limited to 80,000.[2]

This three-tier system of health care delivery helped considerably in developing an infrastructure that would function smoothly if adequate manpower, equipment, materials and medicines were provided, with adequate budgetary support. However, it did not happen this way. For instance, the availability of specialist health manpower in India's health sector indicated an inadequate number of specialists in broad specialties and an imbalance in the rural-urban availability of specialised doctors, with more advanced and specialist physicians and doctors available in the urban areas of the country. As per the norms of World Health Organization (WHO), there must be 25 health workers per 10,000 population, whereas India has only 19 health workers (doctors, nurses, and midwives) per 10,000 population. When we look at the Indian population of more than 1.21 billion, it shows a doctor-population ratio of 1:1700 people against the WHO minimum norm of one doctor for per 1000 population, which is below that of developed countries and some developing countries.[3]

DOI: 10.4324/9781032615660-1

Due to deficiencies in the health care system, poor people in India have been forced to seek health care from the private sector, and often borrow to pay for this health care. Health care has seen a vast improvement over the past decade in India. There has also been emphasis on public-private partnership (PPP) in health care. This is an approach that combines the efforts of public, private and other organisations by contributing to their core competency. It is defined as an arrangement between the public (government) and the private sector in delivering health care services to the citizens. It also provides a means for coordinating with non-governmental agencies to undertake integrated, comprehensive efforts to meet the basic needs of the population and it has emerged as a new path for reforms.

Over the last two decades a majority of the tertiary care institutions in the governmental sector have been facing a resource crunch and have not been able to obtain funds for equipment maintenance, replacement of obsolete equipment, supply of consumables and upgrading the infrastructure to meet the rapidly growing demand for increasingly complex diagnostic and therapeutic modalities. Keeping this in mind, the Ninth Plan suggested levying user charges and establishing pay clinics/pay cabins.

In 1983, the first Health Policy of India was brought out and it was updated in 2002, and again in 2017. The most recent of the four main updates in 2017 mentions the need to focus on the growing burden of non-communicable diseases, on the emergence of the robust health care industry, on growing incidences of unsustainable expenditure due to health care costs and on rising economic growth enabling enhanced fiscal capacity (GoI, 2017). These updates of Health Policies recognised the need for the private health care sector to accomplish the goal of obtaining universal health care as part of Sustainable Development Goals.

According to National Family Health Survey-4, cumulatively, all public sector facilities/providers cater to nearly 53 per cent of the overall health care utilisation across India.[4] Against this, the private sector is being used by 47 per cent.[5] With government expenditure on health as a percentage of GDP low over the years, and the rise of the private health care sector, the poor are left with fewer options than before to access health care services. Thus, public or private health insurance could be a feasible option to overcome excessive out of pocket expenses and possible debt caused to the individual or household in the case of borrowing under catastrophic illness. According to an estimate by the Insurance Regulatory and Development Authority (IRDA) only about 17% of India's population was insured (Mehra, 2016). Thus, using the concept of public-private partnership, the government of India launched schemes aimed at insuring people for health care costs, to avail of health care without undue burden.[6]

In this book we explore various economic aspects of public and private health care delivery, and public and private health insurance schemes, functional in India. This work is divided into seven chapters. The next chapter is about the all India scenario of health facility utilisation, followed by Chapter 3 on sustainable development goals and health insurance in India. Chapter 4 consists of Ayushman Bharat and other state sponsored schemes in India. Chapter 5 deals with the role of public and private sectors in health insurance. This is followed by a look at socio economic correlations of health insurance demand in India. Conclusions and international perspectives comprise the last chapter.

Notes

1 Bhore Committee was set up by Government of India in 1943. It was a health survey taken by a development committee to assess health condition of India. The development committee worked under Sir Joseph William Bhore, who acted as the chairman of committee. The committee consisted of pioneers in the health care field who met frequently for two years and submitted their report in 1946
2 See Annexure Table 1.A.1 to this chapter.
3 See Annexure Table 1.A.2 to this chapter.
4 Within the public sector, a major share of provision of health care facilities has been through three sources which include government/municipal hospitals (22.33 per cent), CHC (14 per cent) and PHCs (11per cent). The remaining public sector providers including government dispensaries, sub-centres, UHC/UHP/UFWC, public Vaidya/hakim/homeopath, ICDS centres, ASHA workers, govt. mobile clinics and others had their individual smaller shares which comprised overall 6 per cent of public sector provision of health care as utilised by the masses.
5 The major shares were from private doctors (27 per cent) and private hospitals (14 per cent)
6 These include RSBY, Ayushman Bharat and a number of State sponsored schemes.

References

Government of India (2017). "National Health Policy 2017" (PDF). Ministry of Health and Family Welfare.
Mehra, Puja (2016, April 9). "Only 17% have health insurance cover." *The Hindu*. Retrieved 18 September 2017.

Annexure

Table 1.A.1 Population norms for Health Infrastructure in Rural India (Public Health Care System)

Centre	Population norms	
	Plain area	Hilly/tribal area
Sub-centres	5000	3000
Primary health centres	30,000	20,000
Community health centres	120,000	80,000

Source: Health and Family Welfare Statistics in India, 2013.

Table 1.A.2 Health Manpower Norms

Country	Physicians per 1000	Nurse and midwife per 1000	Hospital beds per 100,000
Bangladesh	3.6	2.2	6
Brazil	18.9	76	23
China	14.9	16.6	38
Pakistan	8.3	5.7	6
Indonesia	2	13.8	9
Sri Lanka	6.8	16.4	36
South Africa	7.8	51.1	0
India	**7**	**17.1**	**7**
Canada	20.7	92.9	27
France	31.9	93	64
Germany	38.9	114.9	82
Japan	23	114.9	137
Switzerland	40.5	173.6	50
UK	28.1	88	29
USA	24.5	0	29

Source: World Health Statistics, 2015, WHO.

Chapter 2

All India Scenario of Health Facility Utilisation

Evolution of the System

Investment in the health sector in India has been guided by the priorities laid down in each of the five-year plans in the country. Our first national economic planning exercise, viz. the First Five Year Plan (1951–1956), laid emphasis on health-related issues like malaria control, preventive care in rural areas, maternal and child health (MCH) services, family planning and population control and water supply and sanitation. Vertical programmes[1] in the form of separate preventive schemes pertaining to malaria, TB, filariasis, leprosy and venereal diseases were also mooted in the priorities listed in the First Five Year Plan. These vertical programmes and other health sector priorities were again listed in the Second Five Year Plan (1956–1961).

As the health system evolved, the subsequent five-year plans had their own focus. Accordingly, a major shift in focus from preventive programmes to family planning was witnessed in the Third Plan (1961–1966). The strengthening of the rural PHCs and existing vertical programmes became the core focus of the Fourth Plan (1969–1974). A slight shift in the Fifth Plan (1974–1979) occurred with an attempt towards integration of the peripheral staff engaged in vertical health programmes. Further, the Alma Ata declaration in 1978 and ICMR/ICSSR report (ICSSR, 1981) shaped the health sector priorities in later years. These had an impact on health priorities in the Sixth Plan (1980–1984). The Sixth Plan's policy objective was to integrate the development of the health system with the overall milieu of socio-economic and political change in the country.

A major guideline for the health sector in the country evolved with the formulation of the National Health Policy in 1983. This policy reflected the commitment of India to attain the goal of "Health for All by the Year 2000 AD". While emphasising the need for universal, comprehensive and primary health services, the policy document provides a list of goals to be attained by AD 2000. However, achievements were much less than these listed goals.

DOI: 10.4324/9781032615660-2

In the Seventh Plan (1985–1990) and the Eighth Plan (1992–1997) there was a notable shift, with major focus being put on rural health programmes and the private sector's contribution to the health sector. The structural adjustments and less expenditure on health in the initial Plan years coupled with international funding of vertical programmes changed the focus of the five-year plan priorities towards increased private sector participation in the health sector. The subsequent plan periods of 1997–2002 (Ninth Plan) and 2002–2007 (Tenth Plan) emphasised primary care, referral services and decentralisation in the health care sector. In the Eleventh Plan (2007–2012), among the overall 27 national targets, there were four targets for the healthcare sector, which included reduction of IMR to 28, MMR to 1 per 1000 births, TFR to 2.1 and clean drinking water for all by 2009. In the Twelfth Plan (2012–2017), further targets in the healthcare sector included reducing IMR to 25, MMR to 100 and TFR to 2.1. The percentage outlay in the five-year plans in the healthcare sector varies from 3.3 per cent (in the First Five-Year Plan) to 6.5 per cent (in the Eleventh Five-Year Plan) (Table 2.A1.1).

Again in 2002, GOI brought out a new National Health Policy (NHP, 2002) which listed the achievements in the health sector between the years 1951 and 2000. Some of the achievements in terms of major indicators showed a considerable improvement in life expectancy, reduction in crude birth and death rates and infant mortality rate (IMR) as well as a significant improvement in health infrastructure in terms of dispensaries and hospitals, number of beds available and the growth in the number of health personnel, including nurses and doctors, in the country.

Based on achievements so far and keeping in view new threats from diseases like HIV and AIDS, NHP 2002 listed the new goals to be achieved between the years 2000–2015.

Some of the other notable features of NHP 2002 were: the recognition of the need for enhanced health facilities and organisational restructuring of the national public health initiatives to provide more equitable access to health care facilities, emphasis on control of diseases contributing to high mortality (e.g., Malaria, HIV/AIDS) and the need for designing separate schemes tailor made to the health needs of women, children, aged persons, tribals and other socio-economically backward sections of society.

In 2014 and 2017 there were health policies initiated by the government, the former declared a health policy on mental health while the latter focussed on the entire health sector. Some of the main features of this mental health policy are discussed in the section on mental health later in this chapter. However, the main features of Health policy in 2017 are discussed here in this section.

Primarily the National Health Policy, 2017 (NHP, 2017) aims at informing and clarifying the role of the government in shaping health systems in all its dimensions – investments, organisation, prevention of diseases and promotion of good health through cross sectoral actions, access to technologies, developing human resources, encouraging medical pluralism, building a knowledge base, developing better financial protection strategies, strengthening regulation and health assurance.

There are specific Quantitative Goals and Objectives enunciated in NHP 2017. These include broadly three areas, namely, (a) health status and programme impact, (b) health systems performance and (c) health system strengthening.

Thus, some of the major indicators of these are enumerated with quantitative goals. The NHP aims to improve life expectancy and healthy life from 67.5 to 70 by 2025. Following changes in disability index as a measure of burden of disease and its trends by major categories by 2022. It aims for reduction of TFR to 2.1, at a national and sub-national level, by 2025, reduction of infant mortality rate to 28 by 2019, Under Five Mortality to 23 by 2025 and MMR from current levels to 100 by 2020. It also aims to reduce neo-natal mortality to 16 and still birth rates to "single digit" by 2025. It aims for achievement of global target of 2020, which is also termed as target of 90:90:90, for HIV/AIDS, i.e., 90 per cent of all people living with HIV know their HIV status, 90 per cent of all people diagnosed with HIV infection receive sustained antiretroviral therapy and 90 per cent of all people receiving antiretroviral therapy will have viral suppression. Other targets include elimination status of leprosy by 2018, kala-azar by 2017 and lymphatic filariasis in endemic pockets by 2017, elimination status of TB by 2025, reduction in the prevalence of blindness to 0.25/1000 by 2025 and disease burden by one third from current levels. It also envisages to have reduction of premature mortality from cardiovascular diseases, cancer, diabetes or chronic respiratory diseases by 25 per cent by 2025, increase in utilisation of public health facilities by 50 per cent from current levels by 2025, antenatal care coverage to be sustained above 90 per cent and skilled attendance at birth above 90 per cent by 2025, full immunisation of more than 90 per cent of the new born by one year of age by 2025, family planning above 90 per cent at national and sub-national level by 2025, 80 per cent of known hypertensive and diabetic individuals at household level maintaining "controlled disease status" by 2025, relative reduction in prevalence of current tobacco use by 15 per cent by 2020 and 30 per cent by 2025. It also seeks reduction of 40 per cent in prevalence of stunting in children under five by 2025, access to safe water and sanitation for all by 2020 (Swachh Bharat Mission), and reduction of occupational injury by half from current levels of 334 per lakh agricultural workers by 2020.

In order to strengthen the health system, the policy's aim is to increase health expenditure by the government as a percentage of GDP from the existing 1.15 per cent to 2.5 per cent by 2025. It also aims to increase state sector health spending to > 8 per cent of their budget by 2020. It plans to decrease the proportion of households facing catastrophic health expenditure from the current levels by 25 per cent, by 2025. Besides this, the NHP 2017 also aims to ensure the availability of paramedics and doctors as per Indian Public Health Standard (IPHS) norm in high priority districts by 2020, to increase community health volunteers to population ratio as per IPHS norm in high priority districts by 2025, establish primary and secondary care facilities as per norms in high priority districts (population as well as time to reach norms) by 2025. Last, but not the least, it emphasises the development of health information systems and the National Health Information Network by 2025.

Major Challenges

Notably, India has achieved important milestones due to sustained planned efforts. Despite all of the achievements with the prevailing national and state health policies and the systematic five-year plan health sector priorities, there are numerous disconcerting features and newly emerging issues in the health care sector in India. The distressing facts that emerge are: our total population (16.5 per cent of global total population) accounts for one-fifth of the world's share of diseases; a third of the diarrhoeal diseases, TB, respiratory and parasitic infections; a quarter of maternal conditions; a fifth of nutritional deficiencies, diabetes, venereal diseases; and the second largest number of HIV/AIDS cases after South Africa (GoI, 2005).

Besides this high disease burden, the overall state financing of the healthcare sector in India, as noted earlier, has been inadequate, resulting in an unsatisfactory distribution of infrastructure and resources in the healthcare sector. This has led to undesirable outcomes. There is wide-spread disparity in healthcare services in rural and urban areas, poor and rich states and notable neglect of the emerging health needs of the society (Purohit, 2004, 2008). As we adopted a health system based on the recommendations of the Bhore Committee (GOI, 1946), the major responsibility for the health services should have been dependent on the basic infrastructure of public hospitals and PHCs built over the last few decades. However, instead of playing this major role, public sector investment has set up a less efficient healthcare system, thus providing a major impetus to the private sector for an investment which is more inequitable and less regulated. Even the low public investment is largely spent (nearly 70 per cent) towards recurring expenditure (including wages and salaries). Thus, a very small amount is spent on medicines and drugs for patients' care. After taking into account the inflationary factor, real per capita health care expenditure is Rs. 120 only. The overall low spending in the public sector has affected the availability and quality of health care. Based on final outcome indicators, concern is being raised regarding efficient utilisation of this low public sector spending.

Benefits from the public health system have also been uneven across different segments of society. Particularly women, children and socially disadvantaged sections like scheduled castes and scheduled tribes have not received health care in an equitable manner and this is reflected in higher values of IMR for these groups in society.

Moreover, there has been a major policy directive that curative care could be left to the market forces and thus resources could be dedicated to primary care. This is observed in both National Health Policies (NHP, 1983; NHP, 2002). The same emphasis in health policy is seen on the part of the central and state governments that have extended a number of exemptions in the last decade and a half. These have been mainly in the form of excise and import duty exemptions, land subsidy and concessional bank credit. However, this argument in favour of encouragement to the private sector has not really been supported by the recent empirical study based on a sample survey of eight median districts. The study indicates that such a reliance on the private sector, even for curative care, could be contrary to the objective of health policy. Some of the pertinent findings of this survey, for instance, suggest that the private health care is marked by factors like fragmentation of provider market, near absence of private sector providers in the poorest blocks, the overall small size of OPD clinics, urban concentration of these providers, abysmally low per capita ratio of doctors, a high proliferation of technology intensive machines like ultrasound, Doppler machines, CT scans etc., low bed occupancy ratio in relation to public facilities, sub-standard treatment, high cost of care and concentration of three quarters of specialists and technology in few towns (GoI, 2005).

If we presume that the private for-profit sector is going to be a replacement for public sector providers in the delivery of curative healthcare, the findings of this study restrict such optimism and possibly indicate a high cost even in the presence of universal insurance. Given the equity, efficiency and cost implications of sole dependence for health care on the private for-profit sector, it is pertinent to look into the possibility of enhancing efficiency in the public sector or achieving an optimal mix of public and private sector, as well as other alternatives like not-for-profit community-based organisations, to bring better health care facilities to the country.

Financing of Health Care in India

Over a period of time budgetary expenditure in India is much lower than the global average and the average in South Asian nations. This can be observed in Figure 2.1, which presents current health expenditure per capita in US dollars in the years 2000, 2010 and 2016. In 2016, for instance, India's per capita expenditure (62 US$) is much less than China (398 US$), Sri Lanka (153 US$) and Bhutan (91US$).

Likewise, as presented in Figure 2.2, the health expenditure in India as a percentage of GDP in 2016 (4 per cent) is lower than Afghanistan (10 per cent), China (5 per cent), Nepal (6 per cent) and Japan (11 per cent).

Current health expenditure per capita US$

China
398
188
42

Sri Lanka
153
109
44

Nepal
45
30
9

India
62
45
19

2016
2010
2000

Bhutan
91
70
32

Bangladesh
34
20
8

Pakistan
40
27
16

Afghanistan
57
46

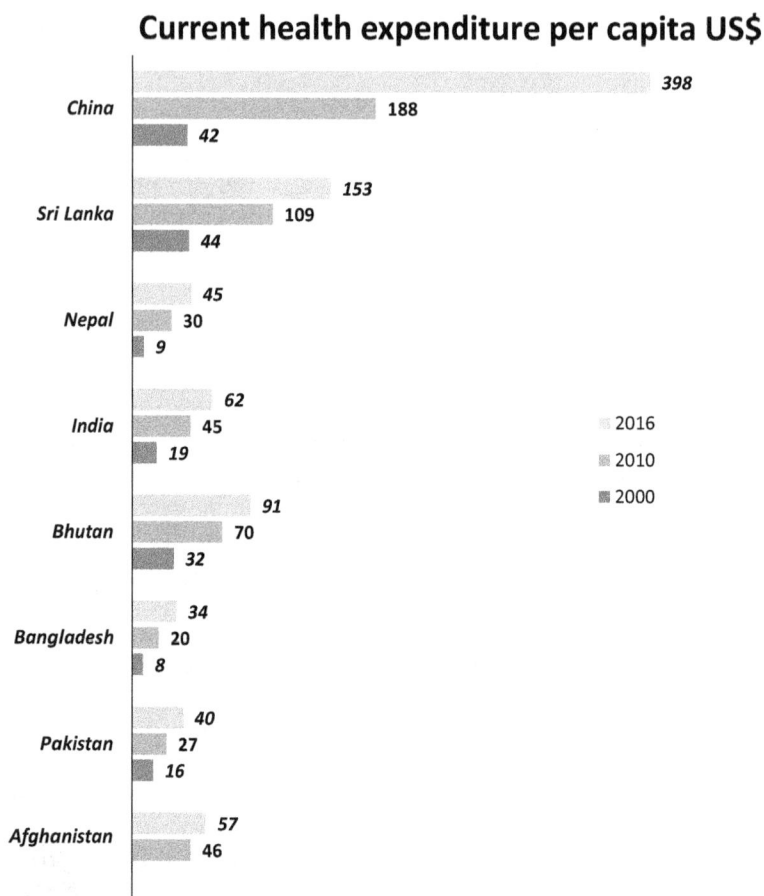

Figure 2.1 Current Health Expenditure in India and Other Southeast Nations (in US$ Per Capita for the Years 2000, 2010 and 2016).

Source: Based on *Global health expenditure*, WHO, 2019, https://apps.who.int/nha/database/ViewData /Indicators/en

It should be noted that current expenditure is not the same as total expenditure. The latter also includes capital expenditure. However, based on National Health accounts (NHA) of Ministry of Health and Family Welfare, Government of India, as presented in Table 2.1 (row 4), we can observe that current expenditures in health have comprised nearly 99 to 94 per cent in the years from 2004–2005 to 2015–2016. This total expenditure is shared largely by the out of pocket expense by the individuals to the tune of nearly 61 per cent (row 6, Table 2.1) and thus the government at different levels in India contributes nearly one third to this total health expenditure (row 5,

Current health expenditure as % of GDP

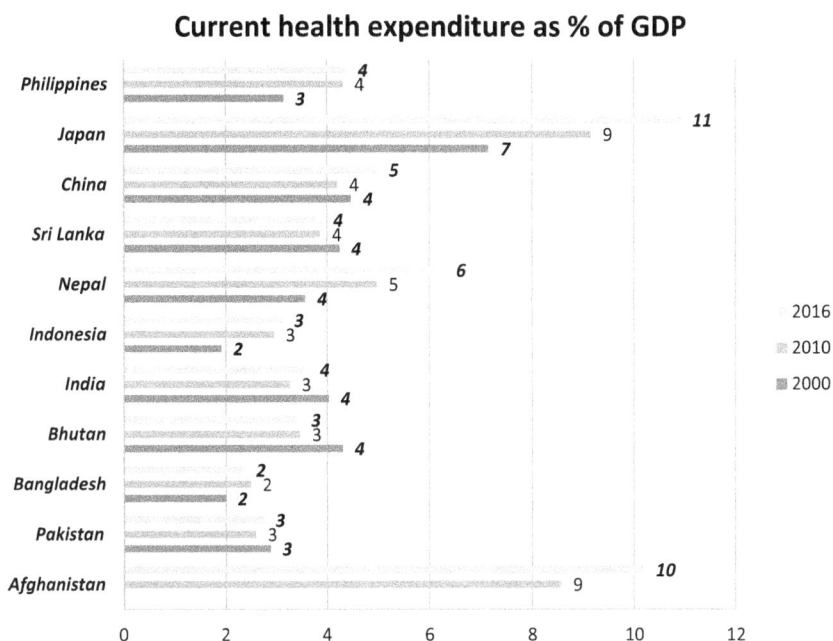

Figure 2.2 Current Health Expenditure in India and Other Southeast Nations (as % of GDP for the years 2000, 2010 and 2016).

Source: Same as Figure 2.1.

Table 2.1).In fact as presented in Figures 2.3 and 2.4, GHE and OOPE comprise 1.18 and 2.33 per cent of GDP respectively and in Rupees per capita the respective amounts are 1261 and 2494 in 2015–2016 (Figure 2.4). In terms of central and state governments and overall insurance through government based agencies they comprise nearly 36, 64 and 3 per cent respectively (Figure 2.5).

The social security (or insurance through budgetary expenditure including health) and private insurance in health only contribute 6 and 4 per cent respectively in the year 2016 (Table 2.1, row 7 and 8). Beside this, very little funds flow to the health sector through foreign aid in India (Table 2.1, last row).

In terms of different health providers as presented in Table 2.2, we can observe that in general, care is distributed across providers including government and private hospitals, private clinics, pharmacies and ambulatory care by the government which comprise nearly 13, 26, 5, 28 and 6 per cent respectively. The remaining percentage of care comprises other types of care or care providers which include specialised care, preventive care, emergency services, medical and diagnostic labs and other agencies' (Table 2.2) terms of

Table 2.1 Key Health Financing Indicators for India across NHA Rounds

Sl. no.	Indicator	NHA 2015–2016	NHA 2014–2015	NHA 2013–2014	NHA 2004–2005
1	Total Health Expenditure (THE) as per cent of GDP	3.8	3.9	4	4.2
2	Total Health Expenditure (THE) per capita (Rs.)*	4116	3826	3638	1201
3	Current Health Expenditures (CHE) as per cent of THE	93.7	93.4	93	98.9
4	Government Health Expenditure (GHE) per cent of THE	30.6	29	28.6	22.5
5	Out of Pocket Expenditures (OOPE) as per cent of THE	60.6	62.6	64.2	69.4
6	Social Security Expenditure on health as per cent of THE	6.3	5.7	6	4.2
7	Private Health Insurance Expenditures as per cent of THE	4.2	3.7	3.4	1.6
8	External/ Donor Funding for health as per cent of THE	0.7	0.7	0.3	2.3

*At current prices. Source: NHA (GoI, 2019).

inpatient and outpatient care and general and specialised care as presented in Figure 2.6, inpatient care constitutes nearly 34 per cent. The same holds for combined general and specialised care. The outpatient care combining general and specialised care comprised 17 per cent of expenditures. The other components include the traditional system of medicines and prescribed medicines. The respective share in expenditures of these components has been observed as 12 and 28 per cent respectively (Figure 2.6).

The segregation of total health care expenditure in terms of primary, secondary and tertiary care is provided in Figure 2.7.[2] It suggests that these three components provide nearly 45, 35 and 15 per cent. respectively, including governmental and private expenditures. Distinction in the latter terms is also shown in the Figure 2.7. It can be observed that the government provided a major share of 51 per cent in primary care in contrast to the private share, which is around 43 per cent. Unlike this, private comprised a major share both in secondary and tertiary care which remained around 40 and 16 per cent respectively. Thus, the role of both government and private provision of care is depicted to be important in the total provision of health care services.

With these shares of public and private care in mind, we now also have a broad pattern of availability of rural health care facilities in India and across

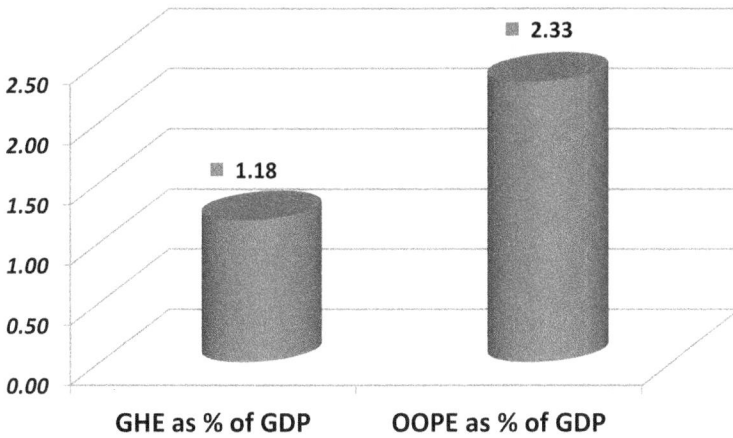

Figure 2.3 Government Health Expenditure (GHE) and out of Pocket Health Expenditures (OOPE) as % of GDP (2015–16).
Source: same as Table 2.1.

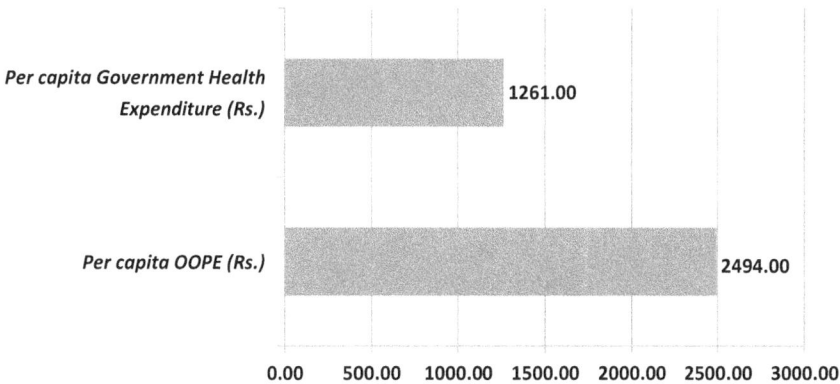

Figure 2.4 Government Health Expenditure (GHE) and Out of Pocket Health Expenditures (OOPE) in Rs. Per capita (2015–2016).
Source: Same as Table 2.1.

major 20 states which include Andhra Pradesh, Assam, Bihar, Chhattisgarh, Goa, Gujarat, Haryana, Jharkhand, Karnataka, Kerala, Madhya Pradesh, Maharashtra, Odisha, Punjab, Rajasthan, Tamil Nadu, Telangana, Uttarakhand, Uttar Pradesh and West Bengal. This is presented in Table 2.3 which indicates a considerable variation across different states pertaining to each of the facilities.

In order to get a better picture, we tried to look into public private shares across two income groups of states. This was based on NSDP per capita in

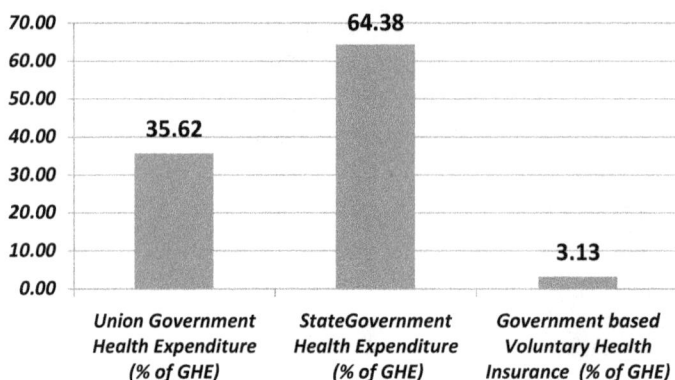

Figure 2.5 Government Health Expenditure (GHE) by Central and State Government and by Govt Insurance.
Source: Same as Table 2.1.

constant (2011–2012 prices) in 2015–2016 which was Rs. 77,659. Focussing on 20 major states, we termed below or above all India income average states which had their per capita NSDP below or above this average in 2015–2016 (see Annexure 1, Table 2.A1.3). Accordingly, the states which were called below all India average income states were Assam, Bihar, Chhattisgarh, Jharkhand, Madhya Pradesh, Odisha, Rajasthan, Uttar Pradesh and West Bengal. The states which were called above all India average states were Andhra Pradesh, Goa, Gujarat, Haryana, Karnataka, Kerala, Maharashtra, Punjab, Tamil Nadu, Telangana and Uttarakhand.[3]

We looked into per capita availability of these rural health facilities (Table 2.4) across Below All India Average States (BAIAS) and Above All India Average States (AAIAS). These are plotted in Figures 2.8–2.12. It can be noticed that in all of these rural facilities there is a pattern which indicates that in BAIAS there is a larger population being served relative to AAIAS. It suggests that there is a difference in availability per capita which is generally lower in BAIAS. This may be due to budgetary funding or other reasons like lower per capita income in these states and thus a lower size of overall budgetary resources.

We also looked into the pattern of total government hospitals as well as rural-urban classifications. This is presented in Table 2.5. There is a lot of variation in terms of average population served by these hospitals across 20 states (Table 2.5). Thus, we further looked into AAIAS and BAIAS (Tables 2.6 and 2.7). There is also a differential across these categories pertaining to government doctors and dental surgeons (Table 2.8) There is indeed a differential pattern across BAIAS and AAIAS in terms of per capita beds available across these facilities. This is presented in Figure 2.13. In line with rural

Table 2.2 Current Health Expenditures (2015–2016)

NHA code	Health care providers	Rs. crore	%
HP.1.1.1	General Hospitals – Government	64,585	13.0
HP.1.1.2	General Hospitals – Private	128,011	25.9
HP.1.2.1	Mental Health Hospitals – Government	1046	0.2
HP.1.3.1	Specialised Hospitals – Government	5323	1.1
HP.1.3.2	Specialised Hospitals – Private	579	0.1
HP.3.1.1	Offices of general medical practitioners (private clinics)	24,488	4.9
HP.3.1.3	Offices of medical specialists (private speciality clinics)	2	0
HP.3.3	Other health care practitioners*** – Government	4196	0.8
HP.3.4.1	Family planning centres – Government	3505	0.7
HP.3.4.9	All other ambulatory centres**** – Government	30,943	6.2
HP.4.1	Providers of patient transportation and emergency rescue	21,604	4.4
HP.4.2	Medical and diagnostic laboratories	22,715	4.6
HP.5.1	Pharmacies	138,061	27.9
HP.5.2	Retail sellers and other suppliers of durable medical goods and medical appliances	792	0.2
HP.6	Providers of preventive care	25,048	5.1
HP.7.1	Government health administration agencies	12074	2.4
HP.7.2	Social health insurance agencies	1662	0.3
HP.7.3	Private health insurance administration agencies	773	0.2
HP.7.9	Other administration agencies	974	0.2
HP.10	Other health care providers not elsewhere classified (N.E.C.)	8809	1.8
	Total	495,190	100

Source: Same as Table 2.1.*** Expenditures on sub-centres/ANM, ASHA, Anganwadi Centres etc. ****Expenditures on Primary Health Centres and Dispensaries including AYUSH, CGHS, ESIS and Railway Polyclinics etc.

health facilities discussed above, there is lower availability and, thus, more population served per hospital beds in BAIAS (Figure 2.13).

We also look into AYUSH system which has been encouraged in the last few years by the budgetary expenditures by both the central and state governments. A synoptic view of availability of the AYUSH system hospitals and dispensaries is presented in Table 2.9. It covers major 20 states. One can notice considerable variations in total as well as individual systems within AYUSH both in terms of hospitals and dispensaries.

However, to get a better picture of the availability of these facilities we present them separately in terms of AAIAS and BAIAS. This is done using the last column of the above Table and also converting to per capita terms

Approximate % of different components in expenditure of health care (based on NHA data)

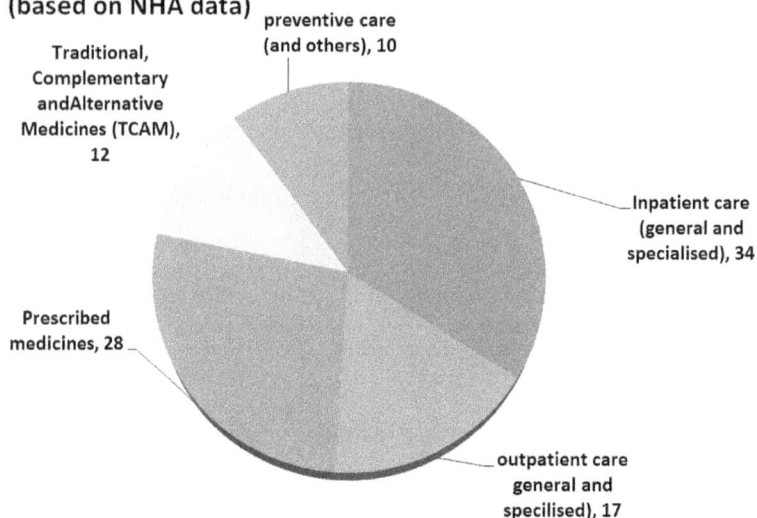

Figure 2.6 Inpatient, Outpatient and Other Components in Health Care Expenditure (2015–2016).

Source Annexure I, Table 2.

by the projected population provided by NHP 2018. These are presented as Tables 2.10 and 2.11 and Figures 2.14 and 2.15 respectively for AAIAS and BAIAS.

If we look at the above Tables 2.9 and 2.10 and compare for AAIAS and BAIAS as shown in Figures 2.14 and 2.15 for per capita availability of hospitals and dispensaries, we observe that AYUSH per hospitals in AAIAS in general has a larger population relative to BAIAS, thus indicating less availability of these hospitals in AAIAS relatively (figure 2.14). However, a similar comparison of per capita dispensaries in AYUSH system as presented in Figure 2.15 indicates that the variations in BAIAS are of a lesser magnitude and availability of dispensaries is relatively lower in AAIAS. Overall, as far as AYUSH system is concerned, there seems to be more liking in BAIAS.

Health Manpower

An overview of health manpower in AYUSH and allopathic systems in India across major states is presented in Table 2.12–2.14. Apparently, there are notable variations across states. In order to get a better view, we provide a comparison across BAIAS and AAIAS in Figures 2.16–2.20. It can be observed that in these health manpower variables BAIAS are generally at a lower level than

Distribution of expenditure across Primay, seconday and tertiery

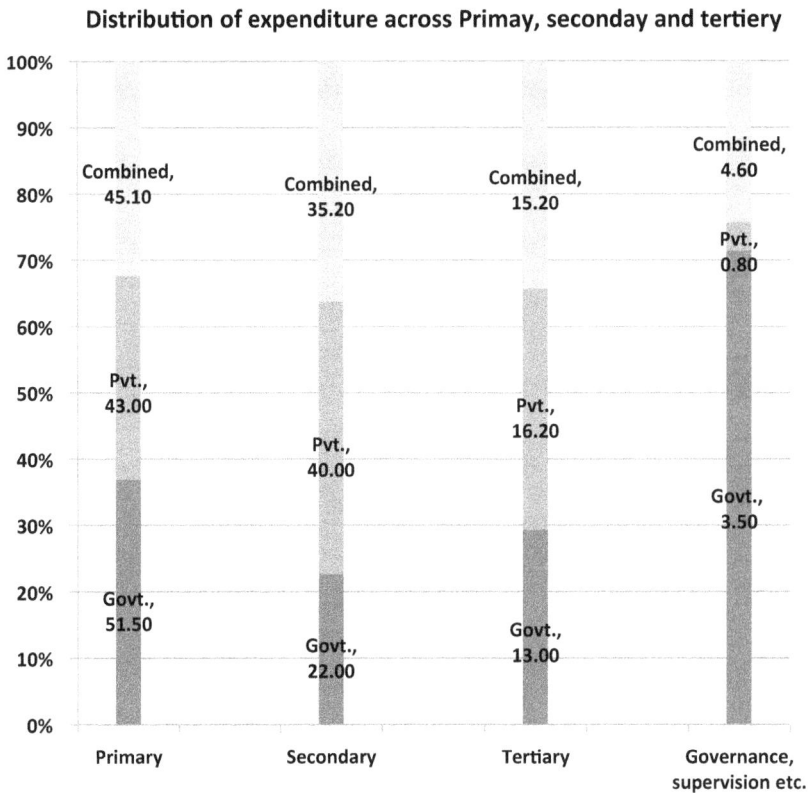

Figure 2.7 Health Care Expenditure across Primary, Secondary and Tertiary Care in India (2015–2016).

Source: Based on NHA data presented in Table 2.A1.1.

AAIAS. Similar indications emerge from Table 2.13 which also depicts other health manpower, namely PHC doctors, CHC specialist, health assistants, LHVs and male/female health workers. Thus, the overall manpower situation for BAIAS and AAIAS suggests the former to be generally below AAIAS.

Mental Health Situation in India

According to National Mental Health Policy of India, 2014 (GOI, 2014) mental health is not just the absence of a mental disorder. It is defined as a state of well-being in which the individuals realise their own abilities, can cope with the normal stresses of life, can work productively and fruitfully, and are able to make a positive contribution to their community. Mental health refers to a broad array of activities directly or indirectly related to

Table 2.3 Rural Health Care Facilities in India across Major 20 States

As on March 31, 2017

States/Union Territories	Sub-centres	PHCs	CHCs	Subdivisional hospital	District hospital
Andhra Pradesh	7458	1147	193	31	8
Assam	4621	1014	158	14	25
Bihar	9949	1899	150	55	36
Chhattisgarh	5186	785	169	18	26
Goa	214	24	4	2	2
Gujarat	9082	1392	363	36	22
Haryana	2589	366	112	21	21
Jharkhand	3848	297	188	13	24
Karnataka	9381	2359	206	146	32
Kerala	5380	849	232	81	18
Madhya Pradesh	9192	1171	309	66	51
Maharashtra	10,580	1814	360	86	23
Odisha	6688	1280	370	28	32
Punjab	2950	432	151	41	22
Rajasthan	14,406	2079	579	19	34
Tamil Nadu	8712	1835	385	279	31
Telangana	4797	689	114	31	7
Uttarakhand	1847	257	60	17	20
Uttar Pradesh	20,521	3621	822	0	160
West Bengal	10,369	914	349	37	22
All India	156,231	25,650	5624	1108	779

Source: https://data.gov.in

mental wellbeing. This is in keeping with World Health Organization's definition of health: A state of complete physical, mental and social well-being, and not merely the absence of disease. Mental health is also related to the promotion of mental well-being, prevention of mental disorders and treatment and rehabilitation of people affected by mental disorders.

Mental health problems refer to conditions ranging from psycho-social distress affecting a large number of people to mental illness and mental disability affecting a relatively small number of people.

Mental illness refers to specific conditions such as Schizophrenia, Bipolar Disorder, Depression or Obsessive Compulsive Disorder.

Mental disability refers to disability associated with mental illness. While mental illness is a medical construct, disability is better understood using a medico-social model and the two terms are not used synonymously. Not all persons with mental illness will have a disability, although many will experience it due to various barriers which may hinder their full and effective participation in society on an equal basis with others.

Both incidence and severity of mental illnesses are on the rise. The World Health Organisation estimates that at any given time 10 per cent of global

Table 2.4 Per Capita Availability of Rural Facilities across Indian States

Population per facility

States/Union Territories	Sub-centres	PHCs	CHCs	Subdivisional hospital	District hospital
Andhra Pradesh	84.404	12.981	2.184	0.351	0.091
Assam	140.841	30.905	4.816	0.427	0.762
Bihar	95.748	18.276	1.444	0.529	0.346
Chhattisgarh	208.198	31.515	6.785	0.723	1.044
Goa	105.783	11.864	1.977	0.989	0.989
Gujarat	144.560	22.157	5.778	0.573	0.350
Haryana	92.276	13.045	3.992	0.748	0.748
Jharkhand	115.893	8.945	5.662	0.392	0.723
Karnataka	137.119	34.481	3.011	2.134	0.468
Kerala	150.797	23.797	6.503	2.270	0.505
Madhya Pradesh	119.773	15.258	4.026	0.860	0.665
Maharashtra	89.168	15.288	3.034	0.725	0.194
Odisha	156.232	29.901	8.643	0.654	0.748
Punjab	100.436	14.708	5.141	1.396	0.749
Rajasthan	197.483	28.500	7.937	0.260	0.466
Tamil Nadu	124.939	26.316	5.521	4.001	0.445
Telangana	126.828	18.216	3.014	0.820	0.185
Uttarakhand	8.340	1.160	0.271	0.077	0.090
Uttar Pradesh	1,954.567	344.890	78.293	0.000	15.240
West Bengal	112.805	9.943	3.797	0.403	0.239
All India	119.174	19.566	4.290	0.845	0.594

Source: Computed based on information from https://data.gov.in and GOI (2018) Central Bureau of Health Intelligence Directorate General of Health Services, Ministry of Health & Family Welfare401 & 404-A Wing, Nirman Bhawan, Maulana Azad Road, New Delhi 110108.

population suffers from some form of mental illness and one in four persons will be affected at least once in their lifetime. Further, estimates suggest that by 2020, depression, the most common mental disorder, will be the second leading cause of disability worldwide, trailing only ischaemic heart disease. The accurate figures for India are not available.

Mental illness is a key predictor for an increase in suicide and suicide attempts that affect a cross section of society, particularly the youth and the distressed. Poverty, deprivation and other vulnerabilities further exacerbate the ground situation.

Untreated mental illness results in stigma, marginalisation and discrimination often worsening one's quality of life. This leads to a substantial loss of social and human capital, adversely impacting a large number of individuals and families.

While the National Mental Health Programme addresses this concern partially, a holistic approach to alleviating distress is necessary. The access to mental health care is not universal, and significant treatment gaps are

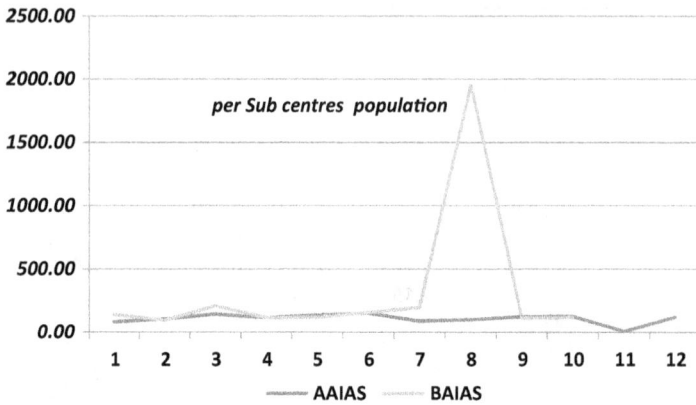

Figure 2.8 Per Capita Availability of Sub-centres in BAIAS and AAIAS.

Source: Based on Table 2.4.

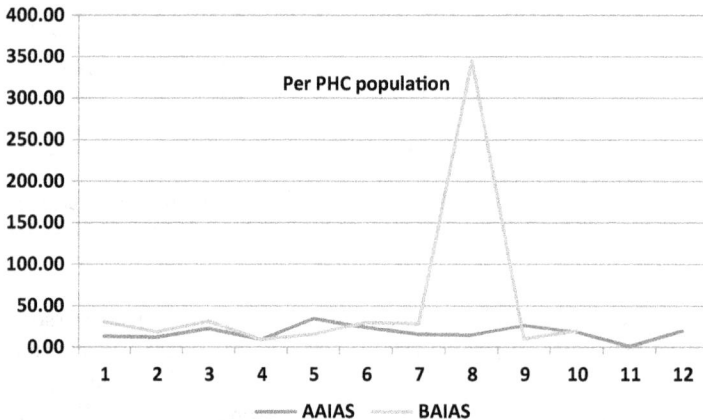

Figure 2.9 Per Capita Availability of PHCs in BAIAS and AAIAS.

Source: Based on Table 2.4.

experienced by many, as a result of which individuals cannot pursue life to the fullest.

Owing to the enormity of the problem, it is considered prudent to have a strategic, integrated and holistic policy that will guide future courses of action including a pan India scaling up of the existing Mental Health Program. This Policy is inclusive in nature and incorporates an integrated, participatory rights and evidence-based approach. Mental health issues are addressed in a comprehensive manner to address medical and non-medical aspects of

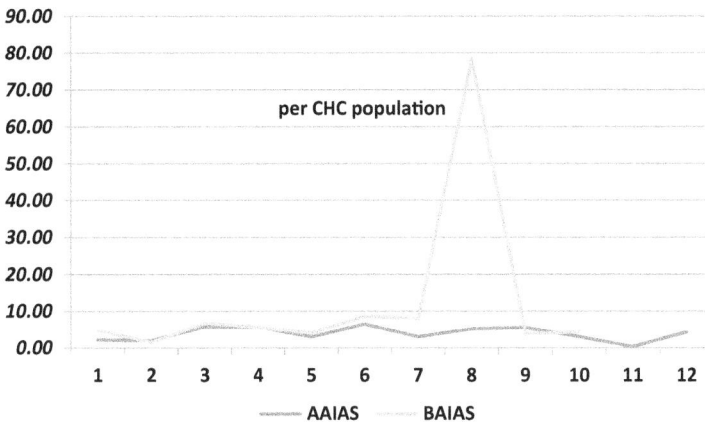

Figure 2.10 Per Capita Availability of CHCs in BAIAS and AAIAS.
Source: Based on Table 2.4.

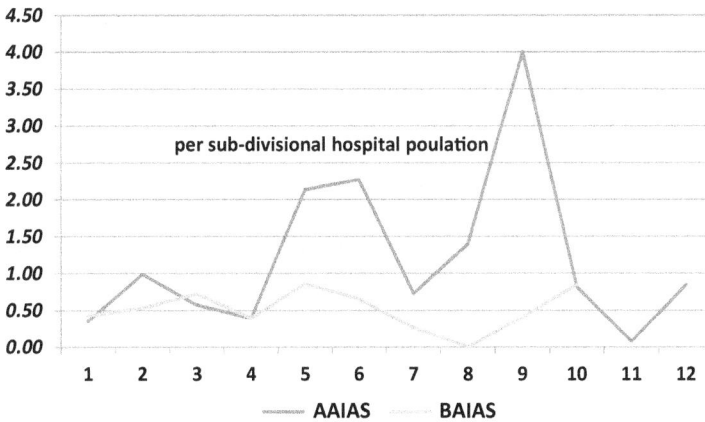

Figure 2.11 Per Capita Availability of Subdivisional Hospitals in BAIAS and AAIAS.
Source: Based on Table 2.4.

mental health. This Policy does not reduce mental health interventions to merely disease and disability prevention and it takes into account the need for all stakeholders to work synergistically and achieve common policy goals.

The strategic areas identified for action are, inter alia, effective governance and accountability, promotion of mental health, prevention of mental disorders and suicide, universal access to mental health services, enhanced availability of human resources for mental health, community participation, research, monitoring and evaluation.

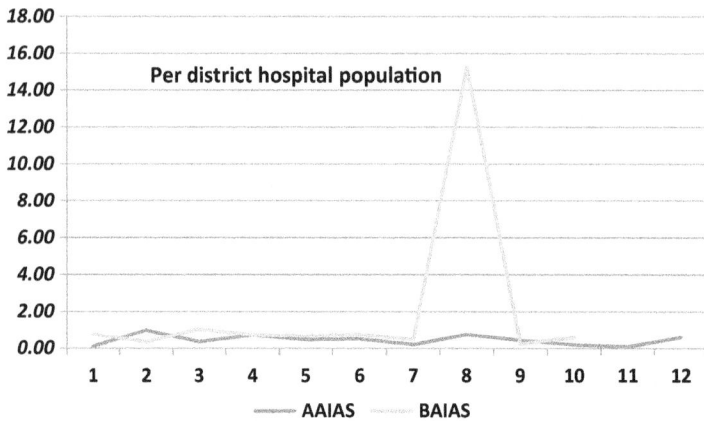

Figure 2.12 Per Capita Availability of District Hospitals in BAIAS and AAIAS.
Source: Based on Table 2.4.

The government believes that mental health is an integral part of our overall health endeavour. A holistic approach that recognises the strong linkage of body, mind and soul is necessary. Strengthening of health infrastructure must be affected, along with addressing the social determinants of health and mental health.

It is significant that the 65th World Health Assembly held in 2013 approved and adopted Resolution WHA 65.4 on global burden of mental disorders and the need for a comprehensive, co-ordinated response from the health and social sectors at the community level. India was one of the main sponsors of this resolution. This National Mental Health Policy is in consonance with the intent of this WHA Resolution Objectives of *National Mental Health Policy of India, 2014:*

To provide universal access to mental health care.

To increase access to mental health care and comprehensive mental health services (including prevention services, treatment and care and support services) by persons with mental health problems.

To increase access to mental health services for vulnerable groups including homeless person(s), person(s) in remote areas, difficult terrains, educationally /socially/economically deprived sections.

To reduce prevalence and impact of risk factors associated with mental health problems.

To reduce risk and incidence of suicide and attempted suicide.

To ensure respect for rights and protection from harm of person(s) with mental health problems.

Table 2.5 Government Hospitals and Beds: Numbers: Rural, Urban and Per Capita Terms

State/UT/Division	Rural Hospitals (Govt.)		Urban Hospitals (Govt.)		Total Hospitals (Govt.)		Projected population	Av pop served per hospital	Av pop served per hospital bed
	number	beds	number	beds	number	beds			
Andhra Pradesh	193	6480	65	16,658	258	23,138	88,361	342,484	3819
Assam *	1176	10,944	50	6198	1226	17142	32,810	26,762	1914
Bihar	930	6083	103	5936	1033	12019	103,908	100,589	8645
Chhattisgarh	169	5070	45	4342	214	9412	24,909	116,397	2647
Goa*	17	1405	25	1608	42	3013	2023	48,167	671
Gujarat	364	11,715	122	20,565	486	32,280	62,825	129,270	1946
Haryana*	609	6690	59	4550	668	11,240	28,057	42,001	2496
Jharkhand	519	5842	36	4942	555	10,784	33,203	59,825	3079
Karnataka*	2471	21,072	374	49,093	2844	69,865	6845	24,056	979
Kerala	981	16,865	299	21,139	1280	38,004	35,677	27,873	939
Madhya Pradesh	334	10,020	117	18,819	451	28,839	76,745	17,0166	2661
Maharashtra	273	12,398	438	39,048	711	51,446	118,652	166,880	2306
Odisha*	1655	6339	149	12,180	1804	18,519	42,808	23,729	2312
Punjab*	510	5805	172	12,128	682	17,933	29,372	43,067	1638
Rajasthan	602	21,088	150	10,760	752	31,848	72,948	97,005	2291
Tamil Nadu*	692	40,179	525	37,353	1217	77,532	69,730	57,297	899
Telangana*	802	7668	61	13,315	863	20,983	37,823	43,827	1803
Uttar Pradesh*	4442	39,104	193	37,156	4635	76,260	221,469	47,782	2904
Uttarakhand	410	3284	50	5228	460	8512	10,499	22,824	1233
West Bengal	1272	19,684	294	58,882	1566	78,566	91,920	58,697	1170
India	19810	279,588	3772	431,173	23,582	710,761	1,310,944	55,591	1844

Source: National Health Profile, 2018, GOI (2018).

Table 2.6 Government Hospitals and Beds: Numbers: Rural, Urban and Per Capita Terms

State/UT/Division	Rural hospitals (govt.)		Urban hospitals (govt.)		Total hospitals (govt.)		Projected population (in thousands)	Av pop served per hospital AAIAS	Av pop served per hospital bed AAIAS
	number	beds	number	beds	number	beds			
Andhra Pradesh	193	6480	65	16,658	258	23,138	88,361	342,484	3819
Goa*	17	1405	25	1608	42	3013	2023	48,167	671
Gujarat	364	11,715	122	20,565	486	32,280	62,825	129,270	1946
Haryana*	609	6690	59	4550	668	11,240	28,057	42,001	2496
Karnataka*	2471	21,072	374	49,093	2844	69,865	68,415	24,056	979
Kerala	981	16,865	299	21,139	1280	38,004	35,677	27,873	939
Maharashtra	273	12,398	438	39,048	711	51,446	118,652	16,6880	2306
Punjab*	510	5805	172	12,128	682	17,933	29,372	43,067	1638
Tamil Nadu*	692	40,179	525	37,353	1217	77,532	69,730	57,297	899
Telangana*	802	7668	61	13,315	863	20,983	37,823	43,827	1803
Uttarakhand	410	3284	50	5228	460	8512	10,499	22,824	1233
India	19,810	279,588	3772	431,173	23582	710,761	1,310,944	55,591	1844

Source: Computed from Table 2.5.

Table 2.7 Government Hospitals and Beds: Numbers: Rural, Urban and Per Capita Terms

State/UT/Division	Rural hospitals (govt.)		Urban hospitals (govt.)		Total hospitals (govt.)		Projected population	Av pop served per hospital BAIAS	Av pop served per hospital bed BAIAS
	number	beds	number	beds	number	beds			
Assam *	1176	10,944	50	6198	1226	17,142	32,810	26,762	1914
Bihar	930	6083	103	5936	1033	12,019	103,908	100,589	8645
Chhattisgarh	169	5070	45	4342	214	9412	24,909	116,397	2647
Jharkhand	519	5842	36	4942	555	10,784	33,203	59,825	3079
Madhya Pradesh	334	10,020	117	18,819	451	28,839	76,745	170,166	2661
Odisha*	1655	6339	149	12,180	1804	18,519	42,808	23,729	2312
Rajasthan	602	21,088	150	10,760	752	31,848	72,948	97,005	2291
Uttar Pradesh*	4442	39,104	193	37,156	4635	76,260	221,469	47,782	2904
West Bengal	1272	19,684	294	58,882	1566	78,566	91,920	58,697	1170
India	19,810	279,588	3772	431,173	23,582	71,0761	1,310,944	55,591	1844

Source: Computed from Table 2.5.

Table 2.8 Government Allopathic Doctors and Dental Surgeons Numbers and Per Capita Terms

State/UT	No. of govt. allopathic doctors	No. of govt. dental surgeons	Provisional/ projected population* as on reference period in (000)	Average population served/govt. allopathic doctors	Average population served / govt.dental surgeon
Andhra Pradesh **	5114	491	52105	10189	106120
Assam	6082	544	32810	5395	60313
Bihar	3576	405	101526	28391	250681
Chhattisgarh	1626	10	25,879	15,916	2,587,900
Goa	521	110	2023	3883	18,391
Gujarat	5475	174	62825	11,475	361066
Haryana	2618	566	26,675	10,189	47,129
Jharkhand	1793	32	33,203	18,518	1,037,608
Karnataka	5047	367	68,415	13,556	186,417
Kerala	5239	172	35,677	6810	207423
Madhya Pradesh	4593	119	78,964	17,192	663,563
Maharashtra	6981	80	118,652	16,996	1,483,150
Odisha	3359	164	42,808	12,744	261,024
Punjab	2992	295	29,372	9817	99,566
Rajasthan	7227	345	79,324	10,976	229,925
Tamil Nadu	7233	584	69,030	9544	118,202
Telangana**	4123	201	38,520	9343	191,642
Uttar Pradesh	10,754	188	214,671	19,962	1,141,869
Uttarakhand	1344	59	10,632	7911	180,203
West Bengal	8829	647	91,920	10,411	142,071
Total	114,969	7239	1,274,095	11,082	176,004

Source: National Health Profile, 2018, GOI (2018).

To reduce stigma associated with mental health problems.

To enhance availability and equitable distribution of skilled human resources for mental health.

To progressively enhance financial allocation and improve utilisation for mental health promotion and care.

To identify and address the social, biological and psychological determinants of mental health problems and to provide appropriate interventions.

Cross-Cutting Issues

Mental health is characterised by cross cutting issues that have a far-reaching impact on the fulfilment of goals and objectives spelt out as policy strategies and need to be addressed through efforts across society. These include (i) stigma, (ii) rights-based approach since violation of their rights is a common reality for persons with mental health problems, (iii) vulnerable populations

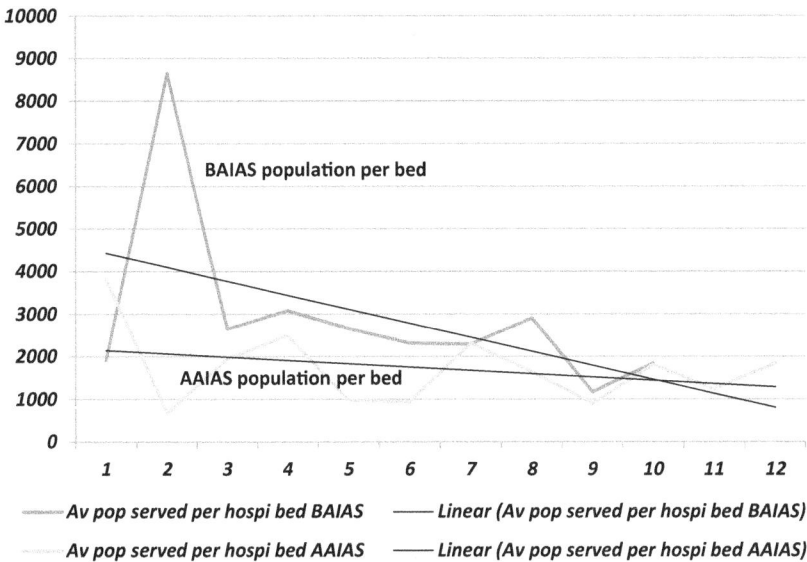

Figure 2.13 Per Capita Availability of Hospital Beds in BAIAS and AAIAS.

Source: Table 2.7.

may include, inter alia, children (both school going and out of school), women, the economically and socially deprived, older persons and persons with physical disabilities. It should be ensured that there is no discrimination against vulnerable populations in the provision of services. Conditions that increase vulnerability and need to be addressed to improve mental health are poverty, homelessness, persons inside custodial institutions and orphaned persons with mental illness (OPMI). It is believed that 70 per cent to 80 per cent of the persons with mental disorders in India live with their families, and this is true across all demographic and social variables. Once the existing caregivers are no more, there is no provision for home care and support of these persons. As a result, many of them languish till death due to starvation and lack of critical support systems like monitoring medicines, personal hygiene and food etc. Not all of them fall under category of poor; yet those with high support needs – irrespective of rich or poor – are highly vulnerable due to their incapacity for self-care. This Policy recognises that the needs of this category of persons with mental disorders have been neglected for a long time, including children of persons with mental health problems, elderly caregivers; elderly caregivers whose own physical and mental health care needs are high and are vulnerable. Unmet needs have a negative impact on their lives as well as the lives of those for who they provide care. There has been little policy or service delivery action to meet the needs of such elderly caregivers.

Table 2.9 Distribution of AYUSH Hospitals and Dispensaries across States and Systems

	Ayurveda		Unani		Siddha		Yoga		Naturopathy		Homeopathy		Sowa-rigpa		Total	
	H	D	H	D	H	D	H	D	H	D	H	D	H	D	H	D
Andhra Pradesh	3	467	2	112	0	0	0	0	0	20	3	266	0	0	8	865
Assam	1	380	0	1	0	0	0	0	0	0	3	75	0	0	4	456
Bihar	5	1082	1	449	0	0	0	0	0	0	2	644	0	0	8	2175
Chhattisgarh	10	956	1	26	0	0	1	0	0	0	3	112	0	0	15	1094
Goa	1	99	0	0	0	0	0	0	0	0	1	83	0	0	2	182
Gujarat	42	560	0	0	0	0	0	16	6	14	16	216	0	0	64	806
Haryana	9	483	1	19	0	0	0	0	0	0	1	22	0	0	11	524
Jharkhand	1	220	0	54	0	0	0	0	0	0	4	92	0	0	5	366
Karnataka	170	592	18	50	1	0	3	0	6	5	16	43	0	0	213	690
Kerala	126	806	0	1	0	6	0	0	1	1	34	659	0	0	162	1473
Madhya Pradesh	21	1496	0	64	0	0	0	0	0	0	2	213	0	0	23	1773
Maharashtra	64	466	6	25	0	0	0	0	0	0	1	0	0	0	71	491
Odisha	8	624	0	9	0	0	0	35	0	30	6	638	0	0	14	1336
Punjab	5	489	0	35	0	0	1	1	1	0	4	111	0	0	9	636
Rajasthan	117	3577	11	120	0	0	0	0	2	3	6	252	0	0	137	3952
Tamil Nadu	2	97	1	64	288	784	1	121	0	0	1	106	0	0	293	1172
Telangana	9	418	4	183	0	1	0	0	1	28	6	196	0	0	20	826
Uttar Pradesh	2104	2104	204	49	0	0	0	0	0	0	8	1575	0	0	2316	3728
Uttarakhand	402	142	2	3	0	0	0	0	0	0	1	60	0	3	405	208
West Bengal	6	502	1	7	0	0	0	0	0	0	15	1520	0	0	22	2029
TOTAL (A)	3165	17128	256	1473	290	815	8	179	17	101	157	7275	0	33	3893	27004
B. CGHS & central government organisation	21	288	8	38	7	33	5	55	2	10	7	269	0	1	50	694
TOTAL (A+B)	3186	17416	264	1511	297	848	13	234	19	111	164	7544	0	34	3943	27698

Source: National Health Profile, 2018, GOI (2018); H=Hospitals, D=Dispensaries.

Table 2.10 Per Capita Availability AYUSH Facilities AAIAS

AAIAS	Per capita AYUSH	
	Hospital	Dispensary
Andhra Pradesh	0.091	9.789
Goa	0.989	89.965
Gujarat	1.019	12.829
Haryana	0.392	18.676
Karnataka	3.113	10.086
Kerala	4.541	41.287
Maharashtra	0.598	4.138
Punjab	0.306	21.653
Tamil Nadu	4.202	16.808
Telangana	0.529	21.839
Uttarakhand	38.575	19.811

Source: National Health Profile, 2018, GOI (2018).

Table 2.11 Per Capita Availability AYUSH Facilities BAIAS

BAIAS	Per capita AYUSH	
	Hospital	Dispensary
Assam	0.122	13.898
Bihar	0.077	20.932
Chhattisgarh	0.602	43.920
Jharkhand	0.151	11.023
Madhya Pradesh	0.300	23.102
Odisha	0.327	31.209
Rajasthan	1.878	54.176
Uttar Pradesh	10.457	16.833
West Bengal	0.239	22.074

Source: National Health Profile, 2018, GOI (2018).

There could be other vulnerable caregivers such as adolescents, single persons responsible for livelihood as well as care giving, and many others such as internally displaced persons. There is a significant demographic shift from rural to urban areas, often across state/regional boundaries. These individuals and families are usually engaged in work in the 0 sector and have poor access to local health services. There is very little information on the mental health needs of this group. Persons affected by disasters and emergencies, other marginalised populations such as commercial sex workers, victims of human trafficking, victims of riot, sexual minorities, children and those living in situations of conflict bear disproportionate burden of mental health problems.

Spending on health by the government is not expenditure but a social investment and a social right. On-going activities under the national and

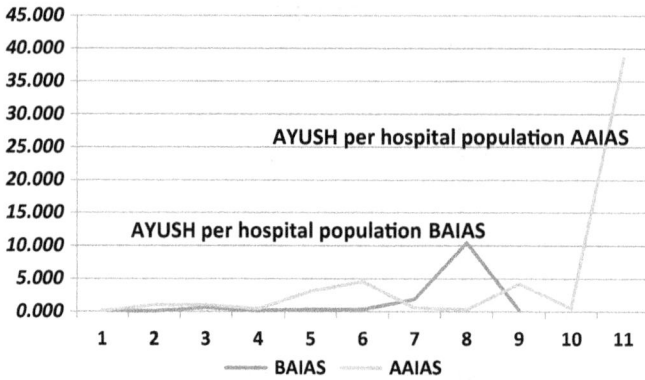

Figure 2.14 Variation of Per Capita AYUSH Hospitals in AAIAS and BAIAS.
Source: Tables 2.9 and 2.10.

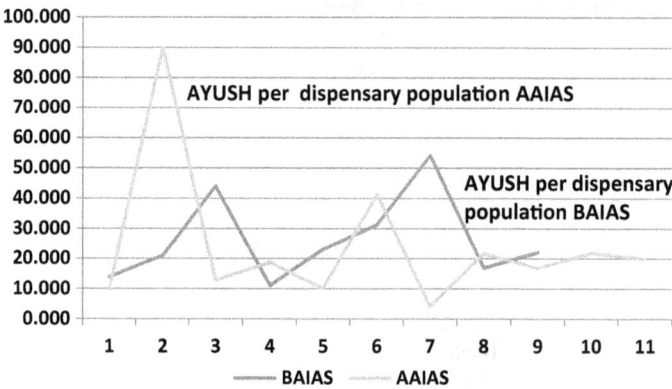

Figure 2.15 Variation of Per Capita AYUSH Dispensaries in AAIAS and BAIAS.
Source: Tables 2.9 and 2.10.

district mental health programmes must continue in a strengthened and more responsive manner. The expansion of the mental health programme to the entire country will require more funds. New activities, especially in the area of community-based rehabilitation and continuing care, must be supported with adequate funding. The work of non-governmental organisations must be encouraged and supported, in order to achieve a collaborative and sustainable response system.

It is also important to keep in mind that additional funding may not be required for many social sector programmes, however, it is imperative to ensure that persons with mental illness are also integrated as beneficiaries of existing programmes.

Table 2.12 State/UT wise AYUSH Registered Practitioners (Doctors) in India as on January 1, 2017

State/UT	Ayurveda	Unani	Siddha	Naturopathy	Homeopathy	Total
Andhra Pradesh	15921	702	0	123	5247	21993
Assam	1002	0	0	0	1160	2162
Bihar	96841	7123	0	0	31992	135956
Chhattisgarh	3430	148	0	102	1824	5504
Goa	636	0	0	0	671	1307
Gujarat	26311	321	0	0	21455	48087
Haryana	8351	268	0	0	5605	14224
Jharkhand	147	30	0	0	285	462
Karnataka	33869	1948	4	745	9102	45668
Kerala	24076	108	1657	147	13156	39144
Madhya Pradesh	46486	1685	0	15	16711	64897
Maharashtra	76465	6833	0	0	64538	147836
Odisha	4846	25	0	0	9645	14516
Punjab	11135	211	0	0	4411	15,757
Rajasthan	9762	983	0	8	7810	18,563
Tamil Nadu	4357	1182	6844	788	5075	18,246
Telangana	10,937	4764	0	314	4809	20,824
Uttar Pradesh	36,626	13423	0	0	33,425	83,474
Uttarakhand	2806	129	0	0	726	3661
West Bengal	3503	5172	0	0	37,178	45,853
Total	428,884	49,566	8505	2242	284,471	773,668

Source: National Health Profile, 2018, GOI (2018)

Currently, families are the main stay of long-term care for persons with mental health problems. Such families bear direct financial costs of treatment as well as associated indirect costs such as loss of wages consequent to having to give up employment to look after sick family members. The emotional and social costs of providing care for a family member with mental illness cannot be quantified but exacts a huge toll on families.

Inter-sectoral Collaboration

Collaboration is also needed within the health sector, for example between specialist mental health and general health services, as well as outside the health sector with education, employment, housing and social care sectors. Similarly, there is need for collaboration between the government (public) sector and the non-governmental sectors (non-profit as well as private).

Institutional Care

Mental hospitals have traditionally been a major source of treatment of persons with mental illness. Over the last few decades, the government has

Table 2.13 State/UT wise Registered Nurses and Pharmacists in India as on January 1, 2017

State/UT Wise Number of Registered Nurses & Pharmacists in India

State	Total No. of Registered Nurses in India as on 31.12.2016			
	ANM	RN and RM	LHV	Pharmacist
Andhra Pradesh	138,435	232,621	2,480	115,754
Assam	27,624	21,079	320	3,668
Bihar*	8,624	9,413	511	4,163
Chattisgarh	13,329	13,048	1,352	9,713
Goa	NA	N/A	N/A	566
Gujarat	44,402	108,476	N/A	119,445
Haryana*	24,675	28,356	694	31,663
Jharkhand*	4,755	3,310	142	2,337
Karnataka*	54,039	231,643	6,840	52,162
Kerala	30,173	246,161	8,507	35,382
Madhya Pradesh*	39,563	118,793	1,731	N/A
Maharashtra	60,837	120,623	572	203,089
Odisha*	62,159	75,575	238	17,665
Punjab*	23,029	76,680	2,584	44,616
Rajasthan*	108,688	200,171	2,732	38,156
Tamil Nadu	56,630	262,718	11,180	58,466
Uttar Pradesh	53,515	62,617	2,763	30,276
Uttarakhand*	1,864	1,513	11	2,643
West Bengal	60,739	60,753	12,854	89,630
Telangana	1,857	4,901	N/A	N/A
Total	841,279	1980,536	56,367	907,132

Source: National Health Profile, 2018, GOI (2018).

undertaken their reform. Even then, their access is limited, staff inadequate and funds low.

Promotion of Mental Health

Key research questions include implementation research issues – how to provide effective treatments in routine health care (for example identification of barriers to integration of mental health into primary health care), causes of mental disorders in the Indian context, identification of effective treatments including those from indigenous systems of medicine which can increase the therapeutic choices for persons with mental health problems, developing a deeper understanding of the bio-psycho-social determinants of mental health and mental illness and pathways for action on the same; among others.

The strategic areas for action are linked to the situation analysis, cross cutting issues and goal and objectives of the Mental Health Policy. Each

Table 2.14 State/UT wise PHC Doctors, Specialist at CHCs and Health Workers in India as on January 1, 2017

	PHC doctors	Specialists CHC	Health assistants Male	LHV	Health worker Male	Female/ ANM
India	27,124	4156	12,288	14,267	56,263	220,707
Andhra Pradesh	1644	348	0	1143	2964	12,073
Assam	1048	139	106	308	2783	9056
Bihar	1786	82	212	95	1244	23,390
Chattisgarh	341	59	425	640	3856	6834
Goa	56	4	0	9	86	195
Gujarat	1229	92	933	1218	7888	8859
Haryana	429	16	153	273	1217	4432
Jharkhand	331	75	33	16	1654	7933
Karnataka	2136	498	3252	1089	3252	7152
Kerala	1169	40	2186	13	3401	7950
Madhya Pradesh	954	180	543	963	3707	11,546
Maharashtra	2929	508	1620	1801	4570	12,135
Odisha	940	318	0	559	3617	8084
Punjab	568	203	268	502	1424	4893
Rajasthan	2382	497	34	1106	1159	16,211
Tamil Nadu	2759	78	1036	991	2109	7957
Telangana	966	125	0	944	1769	7848
Uttar Pradesh	2209	484	13	1916	3835	31,716
Uttarakhand	215	41	954	155	67	2083
West Bengal	918	117	73	157	2174	18,449

Source: National Health Profile, 2018, GOI (2018).

strategic area lists actions to achieve the vision of this policy. Some intervention areas are equally relevant and need to be pursued in parallel. These are: effective governance and delivery mechanisms for mental health, promotion of mental health, prevention of mental illness, reduction of suicide and attempted suicide, universal access to mental health services, improved availability of adequately trained mental health human resources to address the mental health needs of the community, community participation for mental health and development research

The National Mental Health Survey shows urban areas to be most affected (Yasmeen Afshan, 2016). At least 13.7 per cent of India's general population has various mental disorders; 10.6 per cent of them require immediate interventions. While nearly 10 per cent of the population has common mental disorders, 1.9 per cent of the population suffers from severe mental disorders. These are some of the broad findings of a National Mental Health Survey recently conducted by the National Institute of Mental Health and Neurosciences (NIMHANS). That is not all. The prevalence of mental morbidity is found to be very high in urban centres, where there is a higher prevalence of schizophrenia, mood disorders and neurotic or stress-related

AYUSH doctors in BAIAS and AAIAS

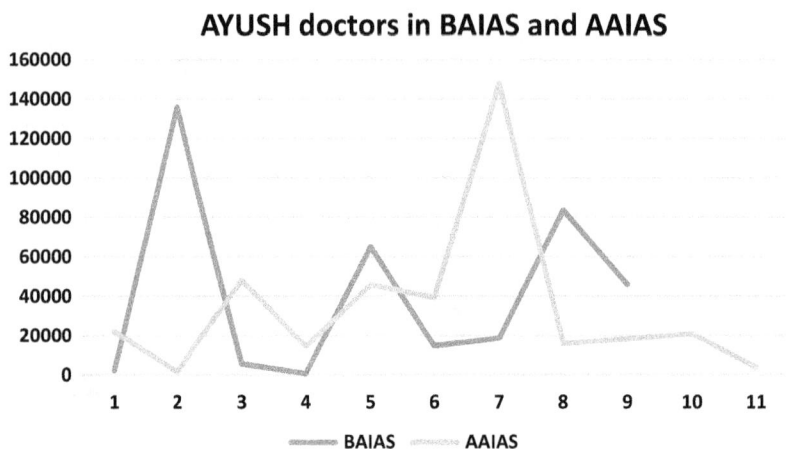

Figure 2.16 AYUSH Doctors in BAIS and AAIAS.

Source: Table 2.11

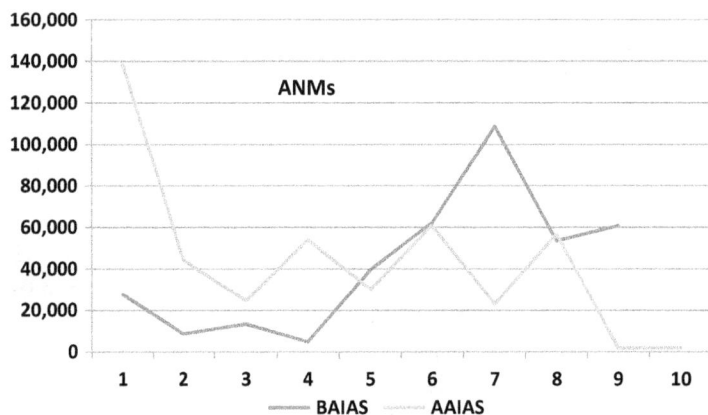

Figure 2.17 ANMs in BAIS and AAIAS.

Source: Table 2.12

disorders. This disturbing scenario could be due to fast-paced lifestyles, stress, complexities of living, breakdown of support systems and challenges of economic instability.

In 2014, NIMHANS carried out a study on mental health status in the country[4]. The study covered all important aspects of mental illness including substance abuse, alcohol use disorder, tobacco use disorder, severe mental illness, depression, anxiety, phobia and post-traumatic stress disorder,

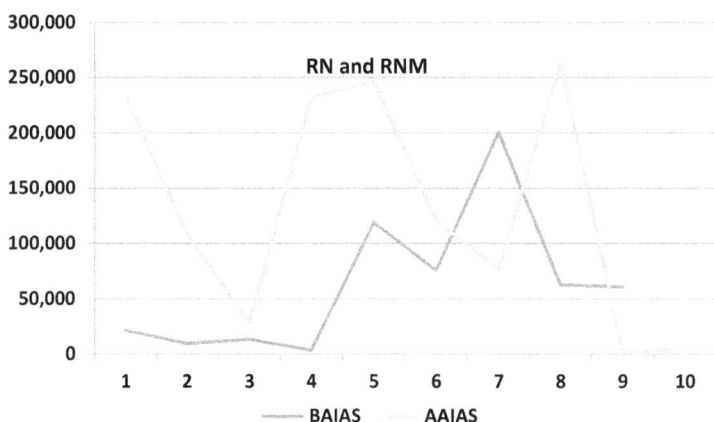

Figure 2.18 RN and RNMs in BAIS and AAIAS.

Source: Table 2.12.

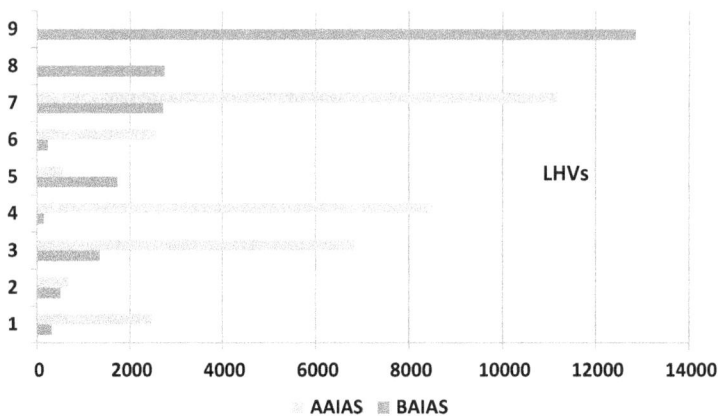

Figure 2.19: LHVs in BAIS and AAIAS.

Source: Table 2.12

among others. It had a sample size of 34,802 individuals. Primary data collection was done through computer-generated random selection by a team of researchers, and local teams of co-investigators and field workers in the 12 states.

While the overall current prevalence estimate of mental disorders was 10.6 per cent in the total surveyed population, significant variations in overall morbidity ranged from 5.8 per cent in Assam to 14.1 per cent in Manipur. Assam, Uttar Pradesh and Gujarat reported prevalence rates less than 10 per

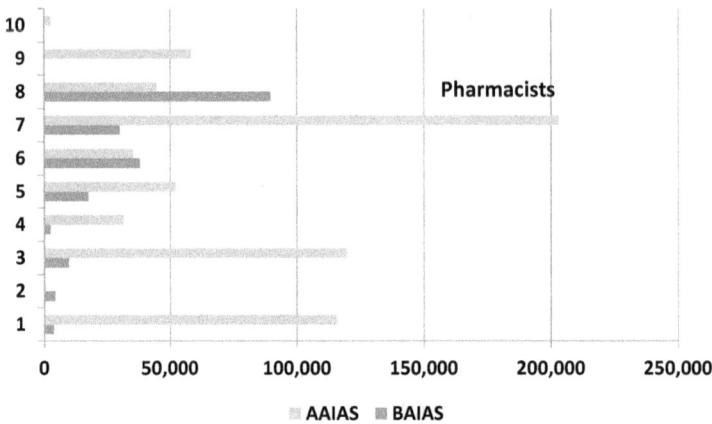

Figure 2.20: Pharmacists in BAIS and AAIAS.

Source: Table 2.12.

Table 2.15 An Overview of Crude Prevalence of Mental Illness and Substance Abuse in India (2015–2016)

Per cent of total respondents	Total respondents (n)↓→ Percentage	Mental morbidity (life time)	Mental morbidity (current)	Intellectual disability (ID)	Tobacco	Epilepsy	Suicidal risk
Assam (AS)	2603	8.14	5.95	0.58	27.78	0.27	5.46
Chhattisgarh (CG)	2841	13.48	11.55	0.60	27.81	0.14	2.18
Gujarat (GJ)	3168	9.31	7.80	0.38	17.96	0.19	4.07
Jharkhand (JH)	3022	11.09	8.57	1.03	10.16	0.43	3.41
Kerala (KL)	2479	14.00	11.21	0.40	7.46	0.36	12.46
Manipur (MN)	2852	19.88	13.85	1.05	20.62	0.35	10.31
Madhya Pradesh (MP)	2621	15.64	12.71	0.84	31.93	0.19	7.25
Punjab (PB)	2895	18.13	13.37	0.48	5.35	0.62	5.18
Rajasthan (RJ)	3108	15.41	11.55	0.45	39.58	0.10	7.95
Tamil Nadu (TN)	3059	19.29	11.80	0.42	8.34	0.26	6.67
Uttar Pradesh (UP)	3508	8.67	6.56	0.46	17.56	0.48	7.10
West Bengal (WB)	2646	15.08	11.83	0.57	13.95	0.04	5.25
Total	34802	13.92	10.47	0.60	19.03	0.29	6.37

Source: NIMHANS (2016).

Table 2.16 Prevalence of Different Mental Disorders

States	Total respondents (n)↓ → Percentage	Moderate	High	Screener positive	Any substance use	Alcohol use	Other substance use	Tobacco use
Assam (AS)	2603	0.6	0.7	0.3	27.3	3	0.7	25.8
Chhattisgarh (CG)	2841	0.4	0.3	0.2	32.4	7.1	1.3	29.9
Gujarat (GJ)	3168	0.4	0.4	0.2	18.8	4.5	0.1	17.4
Jharkhand (JH)	3022	0.6	0.8	0.5	12.8	2.4	0.3	11.9
Kerala (KL)	2479	1	2.2	0.4	10.2	4.8	0.1	7.3
Manipur (MN)	2852	0.9	1.4	0.4	23.8	5.1	0.8	20.7
Madhya Pradesh (MP)	2621	1	0.8	0.2	36.6	10.3	0.6	34.9
Punjab (PB)	2895	0.3	0.5	0.7	11.3	7.9	2.5	5.5
Rajasthan (RJ)	3108	0.7	1	0.1	38.9	2.6	0.5	38.3
Tamil Nadu (TN)	3059	0.3	0.6	0.3	11.3	5.9	0.3	8.2
Uttar Pradesh (UP)	3508	0.9	0.9	0.5	16.4	1.5	0.5	16.1
West Bengal (WB)	2646	1	1.7	0.03	15.7	3	0.8	14.3
Total	34802	0.7	0.9	0.3	22.4	4.6	0.6	20.9

Source: (NIMHANS, 2016).

Table 2.17 Principal Components Using 64 Variables

Number of obs = 12; Number of comp. = 11;Trace= 64;
Rotation: orthogonal varimax (Kaiser off); Rho = 1.0000

Component	Variance	Difference	Proportion	Cumulative
Comp1	11.236	3.552	0.176	0.176
Comp2	7.685	0.832	0.120	0.296
Comp3	6.853	0.253	0.107	0.403
Comp4	6.599	0.483	0.103	0.506
Comp5	6.117	0.662	0.096	0.601
Comp6	5.455	0.436	0.085	0.687
Comp7	5.019	0.514	0.078	0.765
Comp8	4.505	0.478	0.070	0.835
Comp9	4.027	0.515	0.063	0.898
Comp10	3.512	0.517	0.055	0.953
Comp11	2.994	.	0.047	1.000

Source: Estimated.

Table 2.18 Regression result for Moderate Mental Disorder

. reg moderate f4
Number of obs= 12; F (1, 10) = 3.50
Prob> F= 0.0907; R-square = 0.2595
Adj R-squared= 0.185; Root MSE= .25273

moderate	Coeff.	t values	P>t
f4	-.0555	-1.87	0.091
constant	.675	9.25	0.000

Source: Estimated.

Table 2.19 Regression Result for High Mental Disorder

. reg high f1 f6
Number of obs=12; F(2, 9) =5.41; Prob> F=0.0286
R-square= 0.546; Adj R-square= 0.4452; Root
MSE=.41952

High	Coeff	t	P>t
f1	-.0770	-1.84	0.099
f6	.0997	1.66	0.131
constant	.9416	7.78	0.000

Source: Estimated.

Table 2.20 Regression Result for Screener Positive in
            Mental Disorder

Reg screener positive f2
Number of obs=12; F(1, 10)=5.03;Prob> F= 0.0487;
R-square= 0.3348; Adj R-square= 0.2683; Root
MSE=.16281

Screener positive	Coef.	t	P>t
f2	.0397	2.24	0.049
Constant	.3191	6.79	0.000

Source: Estimated.

Table 2.21 Regression Result for Any Substance Use
            in Mental Disorder

reg any substance use f6 f5
Number of obs= 12; F(2, 9)= 3.72; Prob> F= 0.0664
R-square =0.4526; Adj R-square= 0.3309; Root MSE=
8.4229

Any substance use	Coeff.	t	P>t
f6	-2.047	-1.82	0.102
f5	-1.593	-1.50	0.168
Constant	21.291	8.76	0.000

Source: Estimated.

cent. In 8 of the 12 states, the prevalence varied between 10.7 per cent and 14.1 per cent.

A major concern in the findings, which were recently submitted to the Union Health Ministry, is that despite three out of four persons experiencing severe mental disorders, there are huge gaps in treatment. Apart from epilepsy, the treatment gap for all mental health disorders is more than 60 per cent. In fact, the economic burden of mental disorders is so huge that affected families have to spend nearly Rs.1,000-Rs.1,500 a month mainly for treatment and to access care.

According to this study, due to the stigma associated with mental disorders, nearly 80 per cent of those with mental disorders had not received any treatment despite being ill for over 12 months. Poor implementation of schemes under the National Mental Health Programme is largely responsible for this.

There is also a paucity of mental health specialists, pointing out that mental disorders are a low priority in the public health agenda. The health information system itself does not prioritise mental health. It recommended that mental health financing be streamlined, and that there is a need to constitute

Table 2.22 Regression Result for Other Substance Use in Mental Disorder

reg other substance use f3
Number of obs=12; F(1, 10) = 13.86; Prob> F= 0.0040
R-square= 0.580; Adj R-square=0.5389; Root MSE= .44618

Other substance use	Coeff.	t	P>t
f3	-.191	-3.72	0.004
constant	.708	5.50	0.000

Source: Estimated.

Table 2.23 Regression Result for Tobacco Use in Mental Disorder

reg tobacco use f5
Number of obs= 12;F(1, 10)= 4.39; Prob> F=0.0625
R-squared= 0.3052; Adj R-squared= 0.2357; Root MSE= 277.27

Tobacco use	Coef.	t	P>t
f5	-70.846	-2.10	0.063
Constant	552	6.90	0.000

Source: Estimated.

Table 2.24 Regression Result for Epilepsy in Mental Disorder

. reg epilepsy f2
Number of obs= 12; F(1, 10)= 3.33; Prob> F= 0.0980
R-squared= 0.249; Adj R-squared= 0.1748; Root MSE= 4.8452

Epilepsy	Coef.	t	P>t
F2	.961	1.82	0.098
Constant	8.416	6.02	0.000

Source: Estimated.

Table 2.25 Regression Result for Suicidal Risk in Mental Disorder

Reg suicidal risk f3 f6
Number of obs=12; F(2, 9)=13.58; Prob> F= 0.0019
R-squared= 0.7512; Adj R-squared= 0.6959; Root MSE= 42.641

Suicidal risk	Coef.	t	P>t
F3	12.627	2.49	0.035
F6	21.620	3.80	0.004
Constant	184.833	15.02	0.000

Source: Estimated.

Table 2.26 Source of Treatment in India: Public and Private Shares

Source of treatment (all India)	Freq.	Per cent	Cumulative per cent
Public: government/municipal hospital	134,309	22.33	22.33
Public: government dispensary	12,242	2.04	24.36
Public: UHC/UHP/UFWC	6,813	1.13	25.5
Public: CHC/rural hospital/block PHC	85,289	14.18	39.68
Public: PHC/additional PHC	64,290	10.69	50.36
Public: sub-centre	10,293	1.71	52.08
Public: vaidya/hakim/homeopath (AYUSH)	981	0.16	52.24
Public: Anganwadi/ICDS centre	171	0.03	52.27
Public: ASHA	283	0.05	52.31
Public: government mobile clinic	230	0.04	52.35
Other public sector	1,239	0.21	52.56
NGO or trust hospital/clinic	1,925	0.32	52.88
Private hospital	85,381	14.19	67.07
Private doctor/clinic	161,384	26.83	93.9
Private paramedic	5,120	0.85	94.75
Private: vaidya/hakim/homeopath (AYUSH)	1,336	0.22	94.98
Private: traditional healer	2,902	0.48	95.46
Private: pharmacy/drugstore	5,948	0.99	96.45
Private: dai (tba)	102	0.02	96.46
Other private sector	3,484	0.58	97.04
Shop	863	0.14	97.19
Home treatment	870	0.14	97.33
Other	16,054	2.67	100
Total	601,509	100	

Source: NFHS 4 survey (2016).

a national commission on mental health comprising professionals from mental health, public health, social sciences and the judiciary to oversee, facilitate support and monitor and review mental health policies.

While the prevalence of mental illness is higher among males (13.9 per cent) as compared to females (7.5 per cent), certain specific mental illnesses like mood disorders (depression, neurotic disorders, phobic anxiety disorders etc.) are more frequent in females. Neurosis and stress-related illness is also seen more in women. Prevalence in teenagers aged between 13 and 17 years is 7.3 per cent.

Current Situation

An overview of mental illness is presented in Table 2.15. This is based on a survey conducted by NIMHANS in 2015–2016 (NIMHANS, 2016). The total number of respondents in the survey is given in column 1. It is based on nearly 35,000 respondents across the country. However, it suggests that nearly 14 per

Table 2.27 Source of Treatment in India: Public-private shares in Rural-Urban areas

All India Scenario of health facility utilisation (Rural and urban) (NFHS 4)

Where household members generally go for treatment	Freq. rural	Rural per cent	Freq. urban	Urban per cent
Public: government/municipal hospital	78,627	18.48	55,682	31.65
Public: government dispensary	7,741	1.82	4,501	2.56
Public: UHC/UHP/UFWC	4,017	0.94	2,796	1.59
Public: CHC/rural hospital/block PHC	70,205	16.5	15,084	8.57
Public: PHC/additional PHC	57,982	13.62	6,308	3.59
Public: sub-centre	9,668	2.27	625	0.36
Public: vaidya/hakim/homeopath (AYUSH)	655	0.15	326	0.19
Public: Anganwadi/ICDS centre	149	0.04	22	0.01
Public: ASHA	270	0.06	13	0.01
Public: government mobile clinic	163	0.04	67	0.04
Other public sector	556	0.13	683	0.39
NGO or trust hospital/clinic	1,020	0.24	905	0.51
Private hospital	50,786	11.93	34,595	19.66
Private doctor/clinic	1,13,322	26.63	48,062	27.32
Private paramedic	4,371	1.03	749	0.43
Private: vaidya/hakim/homeopath (yush)	985	0.23	351	0.2
Private: traditional healer	2,595	0.61	307	0.17
Private: pharmacy/drugstore	4,555	1.07	1,393	0.79
Private: dai (tba)	71	0.02	31	0.02
Other private sector	2,807	0.66	677	0.38
Shop	684	0.16	179	0.1
Home treatment	642	0.15	228	0.13
Other	13,692	3.22	2,362	1.34
Total	4,25,563	100	1,75,946	100

cent in the country suffer from one of the lifetime mental morbidity whereas the current level of mental morbidity is around 10 per cent (Table 2.15).

A further breakdown of mental disorders in terms of moderate and high and substance use including drug (or any similar kind of substance), alcohol and tobacco is given in Table 2.16. It is notable that nearly one-fifth of the NIMHANS respondents across the country used either tobacco or another addictive substance. However, in states like Rajasthan and MP it was as high as 38.9 and 36.6 per cent respectively (Table 2.16; rows 9 and 7 and column 6). This is followed by Chhattisgarh at 32.4 per cent.

In order to explore the determinants of different mental health provided by the above survey we used socio-economic variables. The information on these variables was also collected by the survey. Mainly these relate to education, occupation, marital status and age groups of the respondents. There are in total 64 variables. The latter include 8 levels of education (including primary, secondary, high school, pre-university, vocational, graduate and

Table 2.28 Source of Treatment in Below All India Average Income States (BAIAS)

combined BAIA states	Frequency	Per cent	Cumulative per cent
Public: government/municipal hospital	10622	15.817	
Public: government dispensary	1102	1.641	17.458
Public: UHC/UHP/UFWC	593	0.883	18.341
Public: CHC/rural hospital/block PHC	16738	24.924	43.265
Public: PHC/additional PHC	8915	13.275	56.540
Public: sub-centre	1641	2.444	58.984
Public: vaidya/hakim/homeopath (AYUSH)	125	0.186	59.170
Public: ASHA	60	0.089	59.259
Public: government mobile clinic	83	0.124	59.383
Other public sector	66	0.098	59.481
NGO or trust hospital/clinic	313	0.466	59.947
Private hospital	470	0.700	60.647
Private doctor/clinic	5541	8.251	68.898
Private paramedic	16046	23.894	92.791
Private: vaidya/hakim/homeopath (yush)	513	0.764	93.555
Private: traditional healer	215	0.320	93.875
Private: pharmacy/drugstore	506	0.753	94.629
Private: dai (tba)	584	0.870	95.499
Other private sector	409	0.609	96.108
Shop	66	0.098	96.206
Home treatment	103	0.153	96.359
Other	2445	3.641	100.000
Total	67156	100	

Source: Computed based on NFHS 4 survey (2016).

post-graduate separately for males, females and across genders). Likewise, the occupation is also classified into eight types (including cultivator, agricultural labour, employer, employee, students, dependents, pensioners and others across male females and all genders separately). The marital status is classified into married, never married, divorcee and widowed (separately across males and females). Age groups are also given in a fivefold category (from one to five). Thus, in order to shorten the 64 variables, we conducted a principal components analysis. This yielded 11 components. Of the latter we used seven components, which explained more than 76 per cent of variation in mental health (Table 2.17).

Looking at the major correlations within each factor derived from principle component analysis (2), we find that factor F1 to F6 respectively largely represent total illiteracy, pre-university education, secondary education, dependent status, female employer and pensioner female.

Using these factors to explain different mental disorders we find that for moderate mental disorders being dependent on others financially acts as deterrent (Table 2.18). However, for high mental disorders literacy acts as

Table 2.29 Source of Treatment in Rural Areas in Below All India Average Income States (BAIAS)

Combined BAIA rural	Frequency	Per cent	Cumulative per cent
Public: government/municipal hospital	6449	12.528	
Public: government dispensary	605	1.175	13.703
Public: UHC/UHP/UFWC	375	0.728	14.432
Public: CHC/rural hospital/block PHC	14535	28.236	42.668
Public: phc/additional PHC	8389	16.297	58.964
Public: sub-centre	1593	3.095	62.059
Public: vaidya/hakim/homeopath (AYUSH)	92	0.179	62.238
Public: Anganwadi/ICDS centre	53	0.103	62.340
Public: ASHA	80	0.155	62.496
Public: government mobile clinic	34	0.066	62.562
Other public sector	65	0.126	62.688
ngo or trust hospital/clinic	140	0.272	62.960
Private hospital	2782	5.404	68.365
Private doctor/clinic	12074	23.455	91.820
Private paramedic	516	1.002	92.822
Private: vaidya/hakim/homeopath (AYUSH)	164	0.319	93.141
Private: traditional healer	494	0.960	94.100
Private: pharmacy/drugstore	511	0.993	95.093
Other private sector	296	0.575	95.668
Shop	60	0.117	95.785
Home treatment	71	0.138	95.922
Other	2099	4.078	100.000
Total	51,477	100	

Source: Computed based on NFHS 4 survey (2016).

deterrent (Table 2.19). But female pensioners seem more vulnerable to this kind of disorder (Table 2.19). This is noted by negative and positive impact coefficient of these variables respectively (Table 2.19).

In case of screener positive mental disorder, pre-university level of education seems to be conducive to its positive impact (Table 2.20). Whereas for any substance use disorder, higher education, female in financially dominating position as pensioner and/or employer seem to be deterrent. It is seen from the negative coefficients of both of these factors (Table 2.21).

In the case of other substance use mental disorder, secondary level education seems to be acting as deterrent and its coefficient represented largely through factor f3 is negative (Table 2.22). Pertaining to tobacco use, status of a female as employer acts as deterrent and its coefficient seen through negative impact of factor f5 (Table 2.23).

Further illnesses like epilepsy also have a positive impact until pre-university education and its impact coefficient as presented largely through F2 is positive (Table 2.24). Lastly the suicidal risk seems to have some positive link and causation through an education level up to secondary and being a

Table 2.30 Source of Treatment in Urban Areas Below All India Average Income states (BAIAS)

Combined below AIA urban	Frequency	Per cent	Cumulative per cent
Public: government/municipal hospital	4173	26.615	
Public: government dispensary	497	3.170	29.785
Public: UHC/UHP/UFWC	218	1.390	31.175
Public: CHC/rural hospital/block PHC	2203	14.051	45.226
Public: PHC/additional PHC	526	3.355	48.581
Public: sub-centre	48	0.306	48.887
Public: vaidya/hakim/homeopath (AYUSH)	33	0.210	49.098
Public: Anganwadi/ICDS centre	5	0.032	49.129
Public: ASHA	2	0.013	49.142
Public: government mobile clinic	9	0.057	49.200
Other public sector	269	1.716	50.915
ngo or trust hospital/clinic	190	1.212	52.127
Private hospital	1745	11.130	63.257
Private doctor/clinic	5041	32.151	95.408
Private paramedic	57	0.364	95.771
Private: vaidya/hakim/homeopath (AYUSH)	61	0.389	96.160
Private: pharmacy/drugstore	104	0.663	96.824
Other private sector	114	0.727	97.551
Shop	6	0.038	97.589
Home treatment	32	0.204	97.793
Other	346	2.207	100.000
Total	15,679	100	

Source: Computed based on NFHS 4 survey (2016).

pensioner, which is noted respectively by the positive coefficients of factors F3 an F6 (Table 2.25)

Health Care Facilities Utilisation: Public and Private Sectors

In this section we analyse healthcare facilities utilisation by patients in either the public or private sector. This is done by using the information provided by NFHS survey (NFHS 4, 2016). Based on this survey, a view of public and private facilities utilisation is provided at all India level in Table 2.26.

It can be seen from the information presented in Table 2.26 that cumulatively all public sector facilities/providers catered to nearly 53 per cent of overall healthcare utilisation across India (Table 2.26, last column). Within the public sector, a major share of provision of health care facilities has been through three sources which include government/municipal hospitals (22.33 per cent), CHC (14 per cent) and PHCs (11 per cent) (column 3, Table 2.26). The remaining public sector providers including government dispensaries, sub-centres, UHC/UHP/UFWC, public vaidya/hakim/homeopath, ICDS centres, ASHA workers, government mobile clinics and others, had their

Table 2.31 Source of Treatment in Above All India Average Income States (AAIAS)

Combined all India above average	Frequency	Per cent	Cumulative per cent
Public: government/municipal hospital	18,254	29.441	
Public: government dispensary	1133	1.827	31.268
Public: UHC/UHP/UFWC	1288	2.077	33.346
Public: CHC/rural hospital/block PHC	4181	6.743	40.089
Public: PHC/additional PHC	6881	11.098	51.187
Public: sub-centre	447	0.721	51.908
Public: vaidya/hakim/homeopath (AYUSH)	97	0.156	52.064
Public: Anganwadi/ICDS centre	8	0.013	52.077
Public: ASHA	13	0.021	52.098
Public: government mobile clinic	25	0.040	52.139
Other public sector	241	0.389	52.527
ngo or trust hospital/clinic	218	0.352	52.879
Private hospital	17210	27.757	80.636
Private doctor/clinic	9696	15.638	96.274
Private paramedic	389	0.627	96.902
Private: vaidya/hakim/homeopath (AYUSH)	76	0.123	97.024
Private: traditional healer	43	0.069	97.094
Private: pharmacy/drugstore	131	0.211	97.305
Private: dai (tba)	16	0.026	97.331
Other private sector	1208	1.948	99.279
Shop	52	0.084	99.363
Home treatment	58	0.094	99.456
Other	337	0.544	100.000
Total	62002	100	

Source: Computed based on NFHS 4 survey (2016).

individual smaller shares which comprised 6 per cent of public sector provision of health care as utilised by the masses. Against this, within 47 per cent share of utilisation by the private providers in all India scenarios, the major shares were from private doctors (27 per cent) and private hospitals (14 per cent) (Table 2.26; rows 14, 15).

However, in order to get a better picture of the utilisation of healthcare across the country we looked in three ways. The latter were looking into the rural-urban scenario separately, poor and rich states separately and rural and urban areas within rich and poor states separately (Tables 2.27–2.33 and Figure 2.21).

As presented in Table 2.27, there is a discernible difference in the pattern of rural and urban healthcare utilisation. While public sector treatment facilities cumulatively catered to 54 per cent in rural areas, it was 45 per cent in their urban counterparts. This indicated more availability and utilisation of private health care facilities in urban areas. The major shares within public sector health facilities for rural population were from government/municipal

Table 2.32 Source of Treatment in Rural Areas of Above All India Average Income States (AAIAS)

Combined above average rural	Frequency	Per cent	Cumulative per cent
Public: government/municipal hospital	11348	27.793	
Public: government dispensary	684	1.675	29.469
Public: UHC/UHP/UFWC	743	1.820	31.288
Public: CHC/rural hospital/block PHC	3418	8.371	39.660
Public: PHC/additional PHC	5908	14.470	54.129
Public: sub-centre	371	0.909	55.038
Public: vaidya/hakim/homeopath (AYUSH)	49	0.120	55.158
Public: Anganwadi/ICDS centre	5	0.012	55.170
Public: ASHA	10	0.024	55.195
Public: government mobile clinic	16	0.039	55.234
Other public sector	125	0.306	55.540
ngo or trust hospital/clinic	115	0.282	55.822
Private hospital	9900	24.247	80.069
Private doctor/clinic	6397	15.667	95.736
Private paramedic	315	0.771	96.507
Private: vaidya/hakim/homeopath (yush)	76	0.186	96.694
Private: pharmacy/drugstore	85	0.208	96.902
Other private sector	953	2.334	99.236
Shop	38	0.093	99.329
Home treatment	27	0.066	99.395
Other	247	0.605	100.000
Total	40,830	100	

Source: Computed based on NFHS 4 survey (2016).

hospitals (19 per cent), CHCs (16 per cent) and PHCs (14 per cent) (Table 2.27; column 3). Comparing this to rural areas, the major share of private facilities utilisation was from private hospitals (12 per cent) and private doctors (27 per cent) (Table 2.27; rows 15–16). In contrast, in urban areas, the major shares of utilisation in public and private facilities were from government/municipal hospitals (32 per cent), public CHCs and PHCs (9 and 4 per cent), private doctors (27 per cent) and private hospitals (20 per cent) (Table 2.27; last column, rows 3, 6–7, 16–15). A synoptic view of this differential pattern is also provided in Figure 2.21.

We expect some difference in the pattern of utilisation between these two groups of states since their per capita expenditures on health by state government are at different levels. A synoptic view of these differences is provided in the Figures 2.22 and 2.23.

As presented in Table 2.28, cumulatively public sector providers in healthcare were a source of treatment for nearly 59 per cent and the private sector was used by nearly 41 per cent in BAIAS. Government hospitals, CHCs and PHCs comprised respectively 16, 25 and 13 per cent in these states. However, unlike all India scenarios, in low-income states private paramedics

Table 2.33 Source of Treatment in Urban Areas of Above All India Average Income States (AAIAS)

Combined above av urban	Frequency	Per cent	Cumulative per cent
public: government/municipal hospital	6906	32.619	
public: government dispensary	449	2.121	34.739
public: UHC/UHP/UFWC	545	2.574	37.313
public: CHC/rural hospital/block PHC	763	3.604	40.917
public: PHC/additional PHC	973	4.596	45.513
public: sub-centre	76	0.359	45.872
public: vaidya/hakim/homeopath (AYUSH)	48	0.227	46.099
public: Anganwadi/ICDS centre	6	0.028	46.127
public: government mobile clinic	9	0.043	46.169
other public sector	116	0.548	46.717
NGO or trust hospital/clinic	103	0.486	47.204
private hospital	7310	34.527	81.731
private doctor/clinic	3299	15.582	97.312
private paramedic	74	0.350	97.662
private: vaidya/hakim/homeopath (AYUSH)	34	0.161	97.823
private: traditional healer	14	0.066	97.889
private: pharmacy/drugstore	42	0.198	98.087
private: dai (tba)	14	0.066	98.153
other private sector	258	1.219	99.372
Shop	14	0.066	99.438
home treatment	28	0.132	99.570
Other	88	0.416	99.986
Total	21172	100.000	

Source: Computed based on NFHS 4 survey (2016).

and private doctors were the major sources utilised by 24 and 8 per cent of population (Table 2.28). A further rural-urban classification of healthcare utilisation patterns by sources of treatment using NFHS survey data is provided in Tables 28 and 29.

It can be observed from Table 2.29 that cumulatively in rural areas public sector provides nearly 63 per cent of utilisation with CHCs, PHCs and government hospitals as major providers at 28, 16 and 12 per cent of share of rural areas utilisation by the people in low-income states. In urban areas in BAIAS, the share of public sector utilisation is lower than rural counterparts at 51 per cent. The major public sector caterers of health care facilities remain respectively as government hospitals (27 per cent) and CHCs (16 per cent) (Table 2.30). Within private sector providers, the main utilisation comes from private doctors (32 per cent) and private hospitals (11 per cent)

The pattern of utilisation in Above all India Average States (AAIAS) can be observed from Table 2.31. Overall public sector provides nearly 52 per cent with a major share in the public sector emerging from government

Source of Treatment (NFHS 4)
(All India-Urban, Rural , Total)(percent)

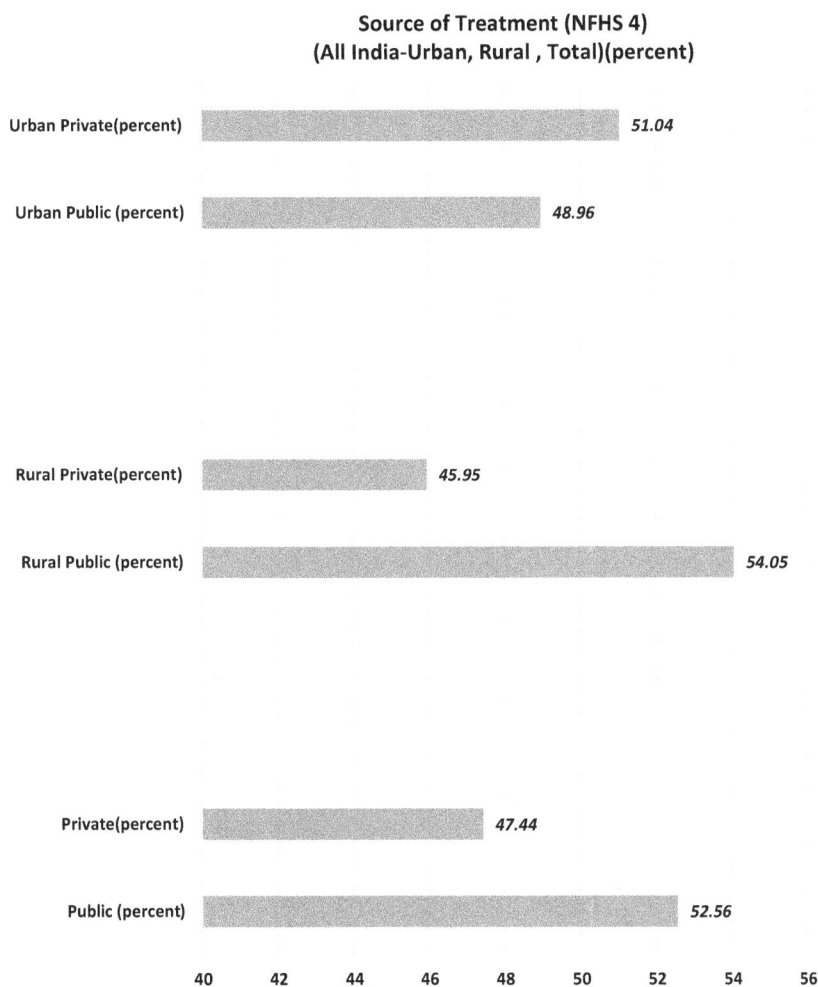

Figure 2.21 Sources of treatment in India: A Synoptic View.

hospitals (29 per cent), PHCs (11 per cent) and CHCs (7 per cent) (Table 2.31). Among major private providers we can observe that private hospitals (28 per cent) and private doctors (16 per cent) are the primes (Table 2.31). In rural areas the pattern in AAIAS suggests that the public sector covers 55 per cent of overall utilisation and major contributors are public hospitals (28 per cent), PHCs (14 per cent) and CHCs (8 per cent) (Table 2.32). Major private providers in rural areas of AAIAS remain private hospitals (24 per cent) and private doctors (16 per cent) (Table 2.32). In urban areas of AAIAS, the

Per capita Health expenditures in Below and above all India average states (2015-16)

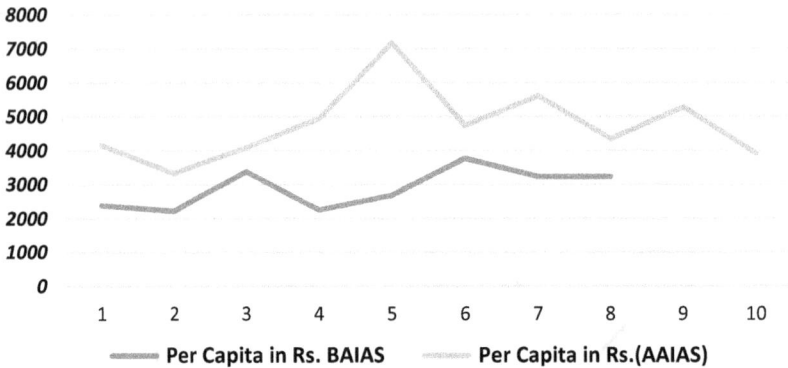

Figure 2.22 Per Capita Health Expenditures on Health in BAIAS and AAIAS.
Source: NHA 2015-16 (Table 3.A.1.1).

Per capita Government health expenditures in Below and above all India average states(2015-16)

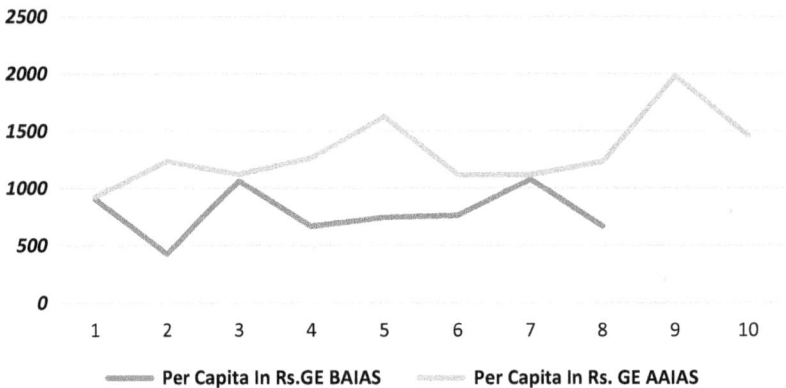

Figure 2.23 Per Capita Government Health Expenditures in BAIAS and AAIAS.
Source: NHA 2015–2016 (Table 3.A.1.1).

pattern of utilisation indicates that the public sector contributes 47 per cent with major providers in the public sector being government hospitals, PHCs and CHCs with their respective contributions at 33, 5 and 4 per cent (Table 2.33). The major contributors to care in private sector in urban AAIAS are private hospitals (34 per cent) and private doctors (16 per cent) (Table 2.33).

Annexure 1

Table 2.A1.1 Five-Year Plan Outlays: Pattern of Central Allocation (Total for the Country & Union MOHFW) (Rs. in crore)

Period	2	Total plan Investment outlay	Health sector	Family welfare	AYUSH	NRHM	NACO	Health research	Total	%outlay
First Plan (1951–1956)	(Actuals)	1960.0	65.2 (3.3)	0.1 (0.1)					65.3	3.4
Second Plan (1956–1961)	(Actuals)	4672.0	140.8 (3.0)	5.0 (0.1)					145.8	3.1
Third Plan (1961–1966)	(Actuals)	8576.5	225.9 (2.6)	24.9 (0.3)					250.8	2.9
Annual Plans (1966–1969)	(Actuals)	6625.4	140.2 (2.1)	70.4 (1.1)					210.6	3.2
Fourth Plan (1969–1974)	(Actuals)	15778.8	335.5 (2.1)	278 (1.8)					613.5	3.9
Fifth Plan (1974–1979)	(Actuals)	39426.2	760.8 (1.9)	491.8 (1.2)					1252.6	3.1
Annual Plan 1979 – 1980	(Actuals)	12176.5	223.1 (1.8)	118.5 (1.0)					341.6	2.8
Sixth Plan (1980–1985)	(Actuals)	109291.7	2025.2 (1.8)	1387 (1.3)					3412.2	3.1
Seventh Plan (1985–1990)	(Actuals)	218729.6	3688.6 (1.7)	3120.8 (1.4)					6809	3.1
Annual Plan (1990–1991)	(Actuals)	61518.1	960.9 (1.6)	784.9 (1.3)					1745.80	2.9
Annual Plan (1991–1992)	(Actuals)	65855.8	1042.2 (1.6)	856.6 (1.3)					1898.80	2.9
Eighth Plan (1992–1997)	(Outlays)	434100.0	7494.2 (1.7)	6500 (1.5)	108 (0.02)				14102.20	3.2
Ninth Plan (1997–2002)	(Outlays)	859200.0	19818.4 (2.31)	15120.2 (1.76)	266.35 (0.03)				35204.95	4.1
Tenth Plan (2002–2007)	(Outlays)	1484131.3	31020.3 (2.09)	27125.0 (1.83)	775 (-0.05)				58920.30	4.0
Eleventh Plan (2007–2012)	(Outlays)	2156571.0	136147.0 *** (6.31)		3988.0 (0.18)				140135.00	6.5
Twelfth Plan (2012–2017)	(Outlays)		75145.3		10044.0	193405.7	11394	10029	300018.00	
Annual Plan (2012–2013)	(Outlays)		6585.0		990.0	20542.0	1700	726	30477.00	
Annual Plan (2013–2014)	(Outlays)		8166.0		1069.0	20999.0	1785	726	32745.00	
Annual Plan (2014–2015)	(Outlays)		8233.0		1069.0	21912.0	1785	713.2	33725.00	
Annual Plan (2015–2016)	(Outlays)		11324.5		1008.0	18295.0	1397	750	30627.50	
Annual Plan (2016–2017)	(Outlays)		14824.6		1050.0	20500.0 #	1700	1500	36374.60	
Annual Plan (2017–2018)	(Outlays)		17661.8		1428.7	27690.7	2000	1800	50281.20	
Annual Plan (2018–2019)	(Outlays)		18570.4		1626.4	32129.6	2100	660	52326.40	

Source: Plan Documents for different plans.

Table 2.A1.2 Current Health Expenditures (2015–2016) by Health care Functions

NHA codes	Health care functions	Rs.Crores	0%
HC.1.1.1	General inpatient curative care	106,941	21.60
HC.1.1.2	Specialised inpatient curative care	63,465	12.83
HC.1.3.1	General outpatient curative care	64,391	13.00
HC.1.3.2	Dental outpatient curative care	369	0.07
HC.1.3.3	Specialised outpatient curative care	20,990	4.24
HC.2	All rehabilitative care	216	0.04
HC.3	All long-term care	20	0.01
HC.4.3	Patient transportation	21,604	4.36
HC.4.4	Laboratory and Imaging services	21,315	4.30
HC.5.1.1	Prescribed medicines	136,364	27.54
HC.5.1.2	Over-the-counter medicines	1697	0.34
HC.5.2.4	All therapeutic appliances and Other medical goods	792	0.16
HC.6.1	Information, education and counselling (IEC) programmes	3824	0.77
HC.6.2	Immunisation programmes	4317	0.87
HC.6.3	Early disease detection programmes	727	0.15
HC.6.4	Healthy condition monitoring programmes	13,832	2.79
HC.6.5	Epidemiological surveillance, risk and disease control programmes	11,239	2.27
HC.6.6	Preparing for disaster and emergency response programmes	94	0.02
HC.7.1	Governance and health system administration	12,646	2.55
HC.7.2	Administration of health financing	2837	0.57
HC.9	Other health care services not elsewhere classified	7508	1.52
	Total	**495,190**	**100**
HC.RI.1	Total pharmaceuticals expenditure (TPE)	175,534	35.4
HC.RI.2	Traditional, complementary and alternative medicines (TCAM)****	58,868	11.9

Source: GoI (2016).

Table 2.A1.3 Primary, Secondary and Tertiary Care Expenditures

	Description of expenditure	Govt	Pvt	Combined
Primary	Expenditures under preventive care under all health care providers.	51.5	43	45.1
	All expenditures at Sub-centres, Family planning centres, PHC, dispensaries (CGHS, ESIS, etc., private clinics) except for those incurred for specialised outpatient care and dental care.			
	Expenditures for general outpatient curative care at all health care			
	providers including related diagnostic and pharmaceutical expenditures apportioned from wherever relevant.			
	Expenditures under all pharmaceuticals and other medical nondurable			
	goods, therapeutic appliances and other medical goods purchased directly by the households			
	Expenditures for inpatient curative care at all ambulatory centres			
	including expenditures related to childbirth at Sub-centres.			
	Expenditures under rehabilitative care at offices of general medical			
	Expenditures under all long-term care and Expenditures under patient transportation			
Secondary	Expenditures under general inpatient curative care at hospitals including related diagnostic and pharmaceutical expenditures apportioned from wherever relevant.	22	40	35.2
	Expenditures under dental outpatient curative care at all health care			
	providers including related diagnostic and pharmaceutical expenditures.			
	Expenditures under specialised outpatient curative care at all providers of ambulatory health care			
	Expenditures under all laboratory and imaging services and pharmaceutical expenditures under specialised outpatient curative			
	care as apportioned from wherever relevant.			
Tertiary	Expenditures under specialised inpatient curative care at all providers including related diagnostic and pharmaceutical expenditures.	13	16.2	15.2
	Expenditures under 0 outpatient curative care at hospitals			
	Expenditures under rehabilitative care at specialised hospitals other			
	than mental health hospitals			
Governance and	All expenditures where both providers and functions are health care	10.7	0.2	3.1
supervision	systems governance and administration of finances			
Not classified elsewhere	Expenditures that could not be classified under any of the above categories	2.8	0.6	1.5

Source: GoI (2016).

Table 2.A1.4 Per Capita Incomes (2015–2016)

S. No.	State	Per capita income 2015–2016 (Rs.) at constant (2011–2012) Prices
1	Andhra Pr.	88,609
2	Arunachal Pr.	84,538
3	Assam	50,642
4	Bihar	23,987
5	Chhattisgarh	61,504
6	Goa	278,601
7	Gujarat	120,683
8	Haryana	133,591
9	Himachal Pr.	112,723
10	J & K	59,924
11	Jharkhand	44,524
12	Karnataka	116,832
13	Kerala	119,665
14	Madhya Pr.	47,763
15	Maharashtra	122,588
16	Manipur	46,389
17	Meghalaya	56,039
18	Mizoram	91,845
19	Nagaland	60,663
20	Odisha	58,165
21	Punjab	100,141
22	Rajasthan	68,596
23	Sikkim	195,066
24	Tamil Nadu	114,581
25	Telangana	112,267
26	Tripura	61,183
27	Uttar Pradesh	36,923
28	Uttarakhand	126,952
29	West Bengal	57,255
30	A & N islands	106,031
31	Chandigarh	197,663
32	Delhi	235,737
33	Puducherry	121,000
34	All India	77,659

Source: (i) Economic & Statistical Organisation, Punjab (ii) Central Statistical Organisation, New Delhi, 2019.

Annexure 2

Table 2.A2.1 Major Correlations in PCA

Variable	Comp1	Comp2	Comp3	Comp4	Comp5	Comp6	Comp7	Comp8	Comp9	Comp10	Comp11
illiteratem	0.231	-0.018	0.005	-0.010	0.099	0.050	-0.001	-0.076	-0.018	-0.040	-0.262
primarym	0.093	-0.187	0.030	-0.194	0.091	0.171	-0.038	-0.007	0.001	0.103	0.042
secondarym	0.067	-0.017	0.283	0.013	0.070	-0.034	-0.086	0.126	0.080	-0.180	0.001
highschoolm	-0.089	0.164	-0.082	-0.085	0.245	0.027	0.038	0.021	0.203	-0.019	-0.100
preunivers~	0.090	0.237	-0.081	0.032	0.079	-0.086	-0.132	0.036	0.059	0.039	0.015
vocationalm	-0.092	-0.066	0.205	-0.089	-0.003	0.050	0.203	-0.279	0.045	0.057	-0.018
graduatem	0.030	0.198	0.041	0.081	-0.217	-0.132	0.105	0.136	0.050	0.158	0.049
postgraduatm	0.102	0.123	0.171	-0.035	-0.209	0.119	-0.041	0.081	-0.091	-0.042	0.005
illiteratef	0.242	0.028	0.025	-0.025	-0.056	-0.022	0.034	-0.001	-0.032	0.077	-0.045
primaryf	0.035	-0.192	0.007	-0.223	0.094	0.152	0.076	-0.011	0.098	0.111	0.148
secondaryf	-0.034	-0.055	0.272	-0.019	0.083	-0.128	-0.117	0.119	-0.021	-0.128	0.122
highschoolf	-0.187	0.115	-0.092	-0.091	0.134	-0.051	0.026	-0.032	0.010	-0.122	0.091
preuniversF	0.031	0.237	-0.108	0.023	0.113	-0.107	-0.142	0.047	-0.053	-0.011	-0.025
vocationalf	-0.145	-0.041	0.164	-0.051	0.019	0.145	0.207	-0.209	0.060	-0.022	0.027
graduatef	-0.178	0.147	0.064	0.026	-0.157	-0.042	0.024	-0.064	0.105	0.055	-0.042
postgradua~	-0.068	0.143	0.169	0.108	-0.178	0.113	-0.055	-0.084	-0.036	-0.119	-0.254
illiteratet	0.245	0.015	0.019	-0.020	-0.008	0.001	0.023	-0.026	-0.029	0.042	-0.113
primaryt	0.066	-0.192	0.013	-0.211	0.093	0.164	0.058	-0.002	0.048	0.108	0.098
secondaryt	0.019	-0.037	0.287	-0.002	0.079	-0.083	-0.103	0.128	0.033	-0.160	0.064
highschoolt	-0.151	0.143	-0.093	-0.093	0.193	-0.017	0.032	-0.008	0.101	-0.079	0.007
preuniverst	0.034	0.246	-0.096	0.029	0.098	-0.099	-0.142	0.045	0.009	0.017	-0.009
vocationalt	-0.108	-0.053	0.199	-0.079	0.002	0.079	0.209	-0.259	0.062	0.010	-0.011
graduatet	-0.085	0.198	0.061	0.060	-0.213	-0.100	0.072	0.038	0.090	0.126	0.011
postgraduat	0.019	0.147	0.187	0.040	-0.216	0.128	-0.052	0.011	-0.074	-0.078	-0.133
malemarital	0.172	0.102	0.135	0.097	0.106	0.077	0.014	0.062	0.161	0.011	-0.107
nevermarried	0.101	0.074	0.054	0.248	0.158	0.130	-0.023	-0.170	0.008	-0.152	-0.143
widowed	0.178	0.086	0.149	0.032	0.007	0.026	0.060	0.173	0.217	0.105	0.044
divorced	0.049	-0.107	0.085	0.049	0.268	-0.112	0.089	-0.118	0.156	0.369	0.213
femalemertal	0.039	0.185	0.201	0.108	0.007	-0.092	0.001	0.024	-0.148	0.000	0.194
fnevermarrd	0.042	0.078	0.011	0.297	0.087	0.026	-0.170	-0.109	-0.213	-0.046	0.263

(Continued)

Table 2.A2.1 (Continued)

Variable	Comp1	Comp2	Comp3	Comp4	Comp5	Comp6	Comp7	Comp8	Comp9	Comp10	Comp11
fwidowed	0.097	0.146	-0.160	-0.086	-0.087	0.169	0.182	-0.030	-0.025	0.067	0.043
fdivorced	-0.143	0.049	0.159	-0.044	0.028	0.149	-0.078	0.162	0.154	0.411	-0.018
firstagegr	0.222	0.071	0.012	0.130	-0.001	0.042	0.011	0.040	0.022	-0.121	-0.021
secongagegrp	0.129	-0.052	0.184	0.049	0.072	-0.199	-0.025	0.207	-0.004	0.217	-0.031
thirdagegr	-0.039	0.063	0.258	-0.007	0.147	-0.064	-0.064	-0.122	-0.020	0.149	0.301
fourthagegr	-0.130	0.113	0.222	0.016	0.086	0.026	-0.064	-0.065	0.030	0.125	0.090
fifthagegr	-0.128	0.204	0.084	-0.027	0.059	0.128	0.101	0.019	0.131	-0.006	-0.153
cultivatorf	0.109	-0.015	0.045	-0.129	-0.276	0.097	-0.069	0.153	-0.181	0.199	-0.155
agriculturF	0.051	-0.135	0.120	-0.214	-0.075	-0.064	-0.197	-0.041	0.051	-0.218	0.285
employerf	0.001	-0.066	0.019	-0.036	0.272	0.292	0.124	0.060	-0.175	-0.002	0.027
employeeotF	0.222	0.090	-0.015	0.016	-0.101	0.013	-0.066	-0.024	-0.021	0.155	0.052
studentf	0.076	-0.164	0.014	0.231	0.043	0.139	-0.053	0.185	-0.078	0.105	0.214
household~	0.203	0.039	0.066	-0.028	0.160	-0.081	0.115	-0.010	-0.110	-0.073	-0.078
dependentf	-0.043	-0.151	-0.051	0.263	-0.057	0.024	-0.077	0.072	0.298	-0.071	0.021
pensionerf	0.064	0.070	-0.069	-0.110	-0.112	0.294	0.113	0.293	-0.037	-0.130	0.214
othersf -	-0.078	0.133	0.172	0.142	0.006	0.169	0.092	0.096	0.199	0.132	0.106
cultivatorm	0.212	0.053	-0.003	-0.095	0.014	0.062	-0.148	-0.180	0.047	0.024	-0.034
agricultur~	0.182	-0.054	-0.018	-0.167	0.044	0.025	0.041	0.070	0.325	0.113	0.132
employerm	-0.051	-0.122	0.195	-0.052	0.198	0.160	0.058	0.095	0.020	0.084	-0.099
employeeot~	-0.113	0.065	0.181	0.180	0.055	0.064	-0.109	0.163	-0.125	-0.115	-0.198
studentm	0.145	-0.172	0.011	-0.143	0.006	0.110	-0.080	0.149	0.144	0.085	0.099
householddm	0.051	-0.089	-0.130	0.154	0.224	-0.089	0.131	0.219	-0.110	0.061	-0.110
dependentm	-0.034	-0.130	0.038	0.256	0.034	-0.141	-0.017	0.151	0.318	-0.050	-0.100
pensionerm	-0.078	0.174	-0.072	-0.025	-0.013	0.156	0.234	0.239	0.033	-0.230	0.073
othersm	0.073	0.037	0.024	0.058	0.017	0.242	0.406	0.017	0.000	0.090	0.023
cultivator~	0.211	0.042	0.007	-0.114	-0.052	0.076	-0.146	-0.126	-0.002	0.066	-0.069
agriculturt	0.149	-0.104	0.048	-0.221	-0.009	-0.014	-0.071	0.026	0.248	-0.036	0.232
employertot	-0.043	-0.118	0.171	-0.050	0.222	0.192	0.074	0.083	-0.011	0.076	-0.088
employeeotot	0.214	0.094	0.060	0.083	-0.056	0.034	-0.093	0.046	-0.066	0.074	-0.037
studenttot	0.123	0.174	-0.012	0.180	0.012	0.122	0.070	-0.165	0.123	0.013	0.134
householddtot	0.201	0.035	0.062	-0.022	0.169	-0.085	0.121	-0.001	-0.114	-0.070	-0.083
dependenttot	0.041	-0.150	-0.034	0.268	-0.042	-0.009	-0.065	0.089	0.311	-0.066	-0.005
pensionertot	0.002	0.130	-0.077	-0.083	-0.081	0.258	0.177	0.294	-0.008	-0.197	0.167
otherstot	0.048	0.004	0.021	0.089	-0.021	-0.266	0.399	0.007	-0.049	0.063	0.044

Source: Estimated.

Annexure 3

Table 2.A3.1 Key Indicators for NHA Above and Below All India Average States (2015–2016)

State	Total health expenditure (THE)			Government health expenditure (GHE)				
	In Rs. crore	Per capita in Rs.	%GSDP	In Rs. crore	Per capita in Rs.	% THE	% GSDP	% GGE
Assam	7874	2386	4	2992	907	38	1.5	7.5
Bihar	24,901	2223	6.5	4756	425	19.1	1.2	4.4
Chhattisgarh	9112	3375	3.5	2871	1063	31.5	1.1	5.6
Jharkhand	7889	2254	3.4	2339	668	29.6	1	5.2
Madhya Pradesh	20,373	2681	3.8	5662	745	27.8	1.1	4.9
Odisha	16,579	3768	5	3354	762	20.2	1	4.4
Rajasthan	23,869	3226	3.5	7980	1078	33.4	1.2	6.2
Uttar Pradesh	69,036	3226	6.2	14,283	667	20.7	1.3	5.2

Table 2.A3.2 Out of Pocket Expenditure (OOPE)

State	Out of Pocket Expenditure (OOPE)			
	In Rs. crore	Per capita in Rs.	% GSDP	% THE
Assam	4339	1315	2.2	55.1
Bihar	19,890	1776	5.2	79.9
Chhattisgarh	5322	1971	2	58.4
Jharkhand	5228	1494	2.3	66.3
Madhya Pradesh	14,283	1879	2.7	70.1
Odisha	11,849	2693	3.6	71.5
Rajasthan	13,455	1818	2	56.4
Uttar Pradesh	52,841	2469	4.7	76.5

Table 2.A3.3 Population, GDP and General Government Expenditure

State	Denominator values (in crore)		
	Population	Gross state domestic product (GSDP)	General government expenditure
Assam	3.3	195723	39702
Bihar	11.2	381501	10,7582
Chhattisgarh	2.7	260776	51646
Jharkhand	3.5	231294	44711
Madhya Pradesh	7.6	530443	11,6606
Odisha	4.4	330874	75896
Rajasthan	7.4	683758	12,8225
Uttar Pradesh	21.4	111,9862	27,7159

Table 2.A3.4 Total and Government Health Expenditures

State	Total health expenditure (THE)			Government health expenditure (GHE)				
	In Rs. crore	Per capita in Rs.	%GSDP	In Rs. crore	Per capita in Rs.	% THE	% GSDP	% GGE
Andhra Pradesh	26,133	4148	4.3	5814	923	22.2	1	5.3
Gujarat	20,990	3332	2	7808	1239	37.2	0.8	6.5
Haryana	11,015	4080	2.3	3033	1123	27.5	0.6	4.6
Karnataka	32,083	4936	3.2	8227	1266	25.6	0.8	6
Kerala	25,090	7169	4.5	5694	1627	22.7	1	6.6
Maharashtra	56,806	4734	2.8	13,443	1120	23.7	0.7	6.3
Punjab	16,234	5598	4.1	3245	1119	20	0.8	6.1
Tamil Nadu	32,975	4339	2.8	9378	1234	28.4	0.8	5.9
Telangana	13,710	5273	2.4	5148	1980	37.5	0.9	5.8
Uttarakhand	4299	3908	2.4	1607	1461	37.4	0.9	5.9

Table 2.A3.5 Out of Pocket Expenses for AAIAS

State	Out of Pocket Expenditure (OOPE)			
	In Rs. crore	Per capita in Rs.	% GSDP	% THE
Andhra Pradesh	19,512	3097	3.2	74.7
Gujarat	10,589	1681	1	50.4
Haryana	6552	2427	1.4	59.5
Karnataka	15,908	2447	1.6	49.6
Kerala	17,889	5111	3.2	71.3
Maharashtra	33,459	2788	1.7	58.9
Punjab	12,563	4332	3.2	77.4
Tamil Nadu	21,500	2829	1.9	65.2
Telangana	7941	3054	1.4	57.9
Uttarakhand	2630	2391	1.5	61.2

Table 2.A3.6 Population, GDP and General Government Expenditure AAIAS

State	Denominator values (in crores)		
	Population	Gross state domestic product (GSDP)	General government expenditure
Andhra Pradesh	6.3	609,934	110,121
Gujarat	6.3	1,025,188	119,948
Haryana	2.7	485,184	66,144
Karnataka	6.5	1,012,804	137,742
Kerala	3.5	557,947	86,190
Maharashtra	12	2,001,223	213,167
Punjab	2.9	391,543	53,133
Tamil Nadu	7.6	1,161,963	159,988
Telangana	2.6	567,588	89,486
Uttarakhand	1.1	175,772	27,304

Notes

1 Starting from the first plan, it was thought that it would take a long time to implement all the recommendations of Bhore Committee, national vertical programmes were started, which later became the centre of focus. These were run and monitored by the Centre. These included Malaria Control Programme, apart from other programmes launched for the control of TB, filariasis, leprosy and venereal diseases. Health personnel were to take part in vertical programmes. However, the first plan itself failed to create an integrated system by introducing verticality. One of the main bottlenecks to the effective delivery of comprehensive health care services at the community level has been the multiplicity of vertical national health programmes. While all these programmes have depended upon the lowly multipurpose health worker (officially called the Auxiliary Nurse Midwife - ANM) for their implementation, the programmes' different planning, monitoring and supervisory systems bring about very uneven pattern of service delivery.
2 Various components included under these categories are described in Annexure Table 3.
3 Key indicators for these two income groups of states are presented in Annexure 3.
4 Concerned over the growing problem of mental health in India, the Union Ministry of Health and Family Welfare had appointed NIMHANS to study mental health status in the country. After a pilot feasibility study in Kolar district, Karnataka, using a sample size of 3,190 individuals, the team began the survey in Punjab, Uttar Pradesh, Tamil Nadu, Kerala, Jharkhand, West Bengal, Rajasthan, Gujarat, Madhya Pradesh, Chhattisgarh, Assam and Manipur.

References

Afshan, Yasmeen (2016, October 23). "India needs to talk about mental illness." *Hindu* op ed.

National Institute of Mental Health and Neurosciences (NIMHANS) (2016). National Mental Health Survey of India, 2015–2016: Prevalence, patterns and outcomes, NIMHANS Publication No. 129, Bengaluru.

Purohit, Brijesh C. (2008). "Health and human development at sub-state level in India." *Journal of Socio Economics* 37: 2248–2260. Elsevier Publications.

Purohit, Brijesh C. (2004). "Inter-state disparities in health care and financial burden on the poor in India." *Journal of Health and Social Policy* 18(3): 37–60. Howarth Press, USA.

Government of India (2002). "National Health Policy 2002". Ministry of Health and Family Welfare.

Government of India (1983). "National Health Policy1983". Ministry of Health and Family Welfare.

Government of India (2017). "National Health Policy 2017" (PDF). Ministry of Health and Family Welfare.

ICSSR-ICMR.3 (1981). Health for all: An alternative strategy. Pune:Indian Institute of Education

Government of India (2005). "National Commission on Macroeconomics and Health (NCMH): Background Papers". Ministry of Health and Family Welfare.

Government of India (2014). "National Health Policy 2015". Ministry of Health and Family Welfare.

Chapter 3

Sustainable Development Goals and Health Insurance in India

Over the past 15 years, the Millennium Development Goals (MDGs) have provided guidelines that relate to various aspects, including health. After analysing the development across the globe and the partial fulfilment of certain goals in different sectors across nations, a new set of inclusive and universal Sustainable Development Goals (SDGs) have been adopted by the United Nations General Assembly in September 2015 as a part of the Post 2015 Development Agenda which came into effect on January 1, 2016. The new Sustainable Development Agenda seeks to ensure that the momentum generated by the Millennium Development Goals is carried forward beyond 2015, to achieve not just substantial reductions in poverty, hunger and other deprivations but finally end them, to provide a life of dignity to all[1].

These goals have also been put in the form of specific targets across various sectors. A list of these targets in the healthcare sector and India's position in achieving these targets is presented below in Table 3.1. We can notice from the S. No. 16 in column 1 that in India we are able to provide essential health services to only 57 per cent of the population as against 100 per cent targets. Also, it not clearly known to us what proportion of the population receives financial protection when using health services. Thus, in this chapter this financial protection or health insurance is our focus.

Further, if we look at the Table 3.2 below, we observe that a large amount of expenditure by the Indian states is being spent in Out of Pocket Expenditure (OOPE) for availing health care facilities.

If we look further at the break up of below all India average states (BAIAS) and above all India average states (AAIAS), we observe that the difference in per cent of GDP between total health expenditure (THE) and OOPE is larger for BAIAS relative to AAIAS. This is indicative of the fact that in poorer states a larger burden is borne by the people in OOPE.

Thus, it is important that we can get a clearer picture regarding availability and utilisation of health insurance and the possibility of mobilising a portion of this OOPE for insuring people's health. In this regard we observe that at present health insurance in the country exists in both public and private sectors.

DOI: 10.4324/9781032615660-3

Table 3.1 Current Status of Health Related SDG Targets – Indian Scenario

S. No.	SDG targets in health	SDG India	Current situation India
1	Maternal Mortality Ratio (per 100,000 live births)	70 per 100,000 live births	174
2	Proportion of births attended by skilled health personnel (%)	To be determined	81.4
3	Under five mortality rate (per 1000 live births)	25 per 1000 live births	47.7
4	Neo natal mortality rate (per 1000 live births)	12 per 1000 live births	27.7
5	New HIV Infections among adults 15-49 years old (per 1000 uninfected population)	0 per 1000 uninfected population	0.11
6	TB Incidence (per 100,000 population)	80% reduction in TB incidence compared with 2015 baseline	217
7	Malaria Incidence (per 1000 population at risk)	90% reduction in malaria incidence compared with 2015 baseline	1
8	Hepatitis B incidence	To be determined	-
9	Reported number of people requiring interventions against NTDs	0	497,396, 247
10	Probability of dying from any of CVD, cancer, diabetes, CRD between age 30 and exact age 70 (%)	1/3 reduction from 2012 baseline	23.3
11	Suicide mortality rate (per 100,000) population)	To be determined	15.7
12	Total alcohol per capita (>15 years of age) consumption, in litres of pure alcohol	10% reduction in harmful use of alcohol	5
13	Road traffic mortality rate (per 100,000) population)	50% reduction	16.6
14	Proportion of married or in-union women of reproductive age who have their need for family planning satisfied with modern methods (%)	100%	63.9
15	Adolescent birth rate (per 1000 women aged 15-19 years)	To be determined	28.1
16	Coverage of essential health services	100%	57
17	Financial Protection when using health services	% of household spending more than 10% on health	-
18	Mortality rate attributed to household and ambient air pollution (per 100,000) population)	To be determined	133.7

(Continued)

Table 3.1 (Continued)

S. No.	SDG targets in health	SDG India	Current situation India
19	Mortality rate attributed to exposure to unsafe WASH services (per 100,000) population)	To be determined	27.4
20	Mortality rate from unintentional poisoning (per 100,000) population)	To be determined	1.9
21	Prevalence of tobacco use among persons 15 years and older (%)	30% reduction in current tobacco use	35
22	Proportion of the population with access to affordable medicines and vaccines on a sustainable basis	To be determined	-
23	Total net official development assistance to medical research and basic health per capita (constant 2014 US$)	To be determined	0.2
24	Skilled health professionals density (physicians/nurses/midwives per 10000 population)	44.5 per 10000 population	30.2
	Average of 13 international Health Regulations core capacity scores	100%	98

Source: Monitoring Health in the Sustainable Development Goals: 2017, World Health Organization, Regional Office for Southeast Asia.

Table 3.2 Total Health Care Expenditure and Out of Pocket Expenses in 2015–2016

State	Total health expenditure (THE)			Out of pocket expenditure (OOPE)			
	In Rs. Crore	Per Capita in Rs.	%GSDP	In Rs. Crore	Per capita in Rs.	% GSDP	% THE
Assam	7874	2386	4	4339	1315	2.2	55.1
Andhra Pradesh	26133	4148	4.3	19512	3097	3.2	74.7
Bihar	24901	2223	6.5	19890	1776	5.2	79.9
Chhattisgarh	9112	3375	3.5	5322	1971	2	58.4
Gujarat	20990	3332	2	10589	1681	1	50.4
Haryana	11015	4080	2.3	6552	2427	1.4	59.5
Jharkhand	7889	2254	3.4	5228	1494	2.3	66.3
Karnataka	32083	4936	3.2	15908	2447	1.6	49.6
Kerala	25090	7169	4.5	17889	5111	3.2	71.3
Madhya Pradesh	20373	2681	3.8	14283	1879	2.7	70.1
Maharashtra	56806	4734	2.8	33459	2788	1.7	58.9
Odisha	16579	3768	5	11849	2693	3.6	71.5
Punjab	16234	5598	4.1	12563	4332	3.2	77.4
Rajasthan	23869	3226	3.5	13455	1818	2	56.4
Tamil Nadu	32975	4339	2.8	21500	2829	1.9	65.2
Uttar Pradesh	69036	3226	6.2	52841	2469	4.7	76.5
Uttarakhand	4299	3908	2.4	2630	2391	1.5	61.2
Telangana	13710	5273	2.4	7941	3054	1.4	57.9

Source: NHA 2015–2016 (GoI, 2016).

Health Insurance Expenditure in the Public Sector in India

Basically, by health insurance we mean any health-financing schemes financed by contributions/premiums collected from individuals or Governments and pooled to actively purchase services from health care providers either by government (health department or government-governed Corporation/Trust/Society) and/or insurance companies.

These schemes could be classified in different government-financed schemes including Social Health Insurance (Central Government Health Scheme, Employees' State Insurance Scheme and Ex-Servicemen Contributory Health Scheme), Government Financed Health Insurance Schemes (of both union and state governments), employer-based insurance – other than enterprises schemes (Private Group Health Insurance), other primary coverage schemes (Private Individual Health Insurance) and community-based health insurance (NPH, 2018).

Also within government-financed insurance schemes, as depicted in the budgetary statements, insurance expenditures do not include (1) medical reimbursements to union government employees reported under Central Services Medical Attendance (CSMA), expenditures on health care services provided by Defence and Railways (2) state government reimbursement of medical bills to its employees (3) union and state governments' medical relief or medical emergency funds released on specific individual requests to below poverty line and vulnerable populations for secondary and tertiary care. As per SHA 2011 and NHA Guidelines for India 2016, expenditures under (1) & (2) are included under union and state government employee schemes and expenditures under (3) are included under union and state government non-employee schemes.[2]

Thus, the expenditures in terms of percentages to total health insurance expenditure in India in 2015–2016 is depicted in three broad categories namely

Table 3.3 Difference in Per cent GDP of THE and OOPE

BAIAS	AAIAS
0.55	0.74
0.80	0.50
0.57	0.61
0.68	0.50
0.71	0.71
0.72	0.61
0.57	0.78
0.76	0.68
	0.63
	0.58
.55-.80	.50-.78

Source: NHA 2015–2016 (GoI, 2016).

social, government-financed and private health insurance in Figure 3.1. This indicates that at present the share of public and private health insurance is 51:49. It also depicts that the three schemes which fall under social health insurance, namely central government health insurance scheme (CGHS), Employees State Insurance Scheme (ESIS) and Ex-Serviceman Contributory Health Scheme are the only ones which may be classified as social health insurance. The distinction between a health insurance and social health insurance is that the latter also provides for compensation for lost wages due to absence of work due to sickness, maternity and/or partial disability by loss of a limb and death due to injury at work to workers. However, these items in the NHA are not included. Thus our Figure 3.1 also does not include such items.

Table 3.4 below presents an estimate of expenditures incurred by the central and state governments under various health insurance schemes as well as the individuals in the country.

It is interesting to note from Table 3.4 that there are as many as 22 health insurance schemes that are also functioning as public sector government-financed schemes.

In this section we focus on two of the social insurance schemes, namely, CGHS and ESIS

Central Government Health Insurance Scheme (CGHS)

The Central Government Health Scheme (CGHS) is a health scheme for serving/retired Central Government employees and their families. CGHS has a beneficiary base of 3,247,783 members and it comprises serving employees, pensioners, Members of Parliament (present and past), freedom fighters and others.

Subscription rates for CGHS membership: this ranges between Rs 50 to Rs 500 depending on the Grade pay drawn.

Facilities available to CGHS beneficiaries at present are –

1. OPD treatment and medicines from CGHS Wellness Centres.
2. Hospitalisation at Government and CGHS empanelled hospitals.
3. Investigations at Government and empanelled Diagnostic centres.
4. Specialist Consultation at Government Hospitals.
5. Beneficiaries can go to any CGHS Wellness Centre in the country.
6. Reimbursement of expenses incurred for purchase of Hearing Aid, Hip/Knee Joint implants, Artificial Limbs, Pacemakers, ICD/Combo device, CPAP, BiPAP, Oxygen Concentrator etc., as per the CGHS ceiling rates and guidelines.
7. In case of emergency, CGHS beneficiaries can go to any hospital, empanelled or non-empanelled and avail of medical treatment.
8. In case of emergency there is provision of reimbursement of expenses for treatment in private unrecognised hospitals

Expenditure under Three Catogries of Health Insurances in India (in% ; 2015-16)

Private Health Insurance — 51.23

Government Financed Health Insurance — 11.79

Social Health Insurance Schemes — 36.98

0.00   10.00   20.00   30.00   40.00   50.00   60.00

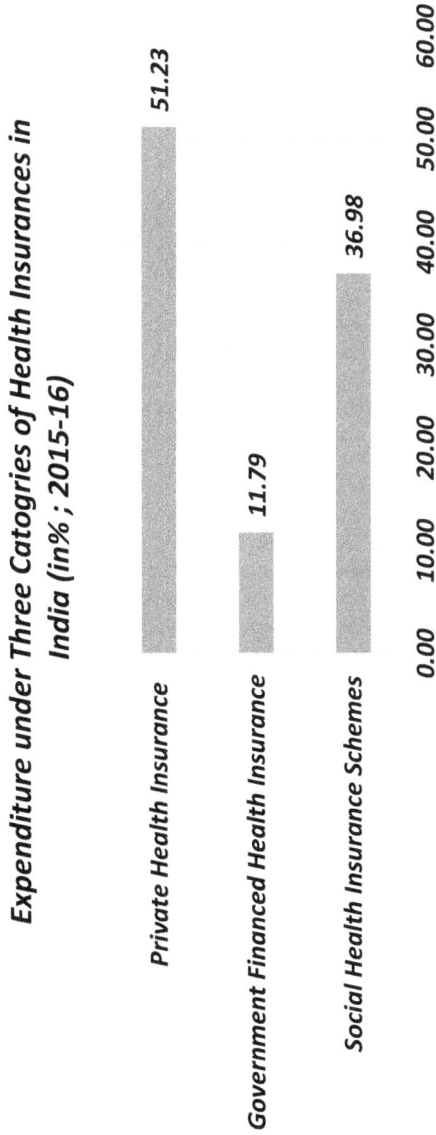

Figure 3.1 Expenditures among Three Broad Health Insurances in India.

Source: Estimated.

Table 3.4 Health Insurance Expenditure (2015–2016) under Different Schemes

NHA Codes	Health insurance scheme	Rs. crore
1	Social Health Insurance Schemes	15,889
1.1	Central Government Health Scheme (CGHS) (Incl. Capital Expenditure of Rs.28 Cr	2913
1.2	Employee State Insurance Scheme (ESIS) (Incl. Capital Expenditure of Rs.114.56 Cr)	10,413
1.3	Ex-Serviceman Contributory Health Scheme Incl. Capital Expenditure of Rs.5 Cr)	2563
2	Government-Financed Health Insurance	5064
2.1	Rashtriya Swasthya Bima Yojana (RSBY) (All States Not Specified Else Where)	1171
2.2	Comprehensive Health Insurance, Arunachal Pradesh	17
2.3	Yeshasvini Health Insurance, Karnataka	285
2.4	Aarogyasri Health Insurance, Telangana	437
2.5	Handloom Weaver Health Insurance	20
2.6	Insurance for Information and Broadcasting Workers, West Bengal	2
2.7	NTR Vaidyaseva, Andhra Pradesh	620
2.8	Chief Minister's Health Insurance Scheme, Chhattisgarh	38
2.9	Goa Mediclaim and Swarnjayanti Aarogya Bima Yojna, Goa	10
2.10	Mukhyamantri Amrutam Yojna, Gujarat	118
2.11	Mukhya Mantri Health Insurance, Himachal Pradesh	2
2.12	Suvarna Arogya Suraksha Trust, Karnataka***	178
2.13	Mahatama Jyotiba Phule Jan Arogya Yojana, Maharashtra	868
2.14	Megha Health Insurance, Meghalaya (Incl. RSBY)	25
2.15	Public Health Insurance, Mizoram	9
2.16	Bhagat Puran Singh Health Insurance Punjab	18
2.17	Chief Minister's Health Insurance, Tamil Nadu	953
2.18	Chief Minister Swasthya BimaYojna Uttarakhand	24.5
2.19	Pradhan Mantri Swasthya Suraksha Yojna Puducherry (Incl. Assistance for Poor through Medical Relief Society)	8.5
2.20	Biju Krushak Yojana, Odisha	100
2.21	Comprehensive Health Insurance Scheme, Kerala	154
2.22	Other Government-Financed Health Insurance****	5
3	Private Health Insurance	22,013
3.1	Employer-based insurance (Other than enterprises schemes)	11621
3.2	Other primary coverage schemes	10,353
3.3	Community-based insurance	39

Note: All values in the above table are rounded off*** Suvarna Aarogya Suraksha Trust is an institution that manages several schemes that provide cashless health care services to entitled households and reimburse directly to health care providers wherein all expenditures are largely financed by the state government of Karnataka.**** There are some small insurance schemes reported by Union Ministries, Urban Local bodies or state governments which are specific to certain occupation group or poor/ vulnerable populations. Such schemes have no specific name and have small expenditures. Also, these may be one with no promise to continue in the future. Thus, these are not presented independently and summed up under this head.

9. Medical consultation and dispensing of medicines in Ayurveda, Homeopathy, Unani and Siddha systems of medicine (AYUSH).
10. Issue of Medicines for up to three months in respect of treatment of chronic illnesses on the basis of valid prescription of Government Specialist.
11. Pensioners and other identified beneficiaries have facilities for cash-less treatment in empanelled hospitals and diagnostic centres; Family Welfare & MCH Services.

Expenditure on CGHS

Between 2011–2017 the total expenditure has grown from Rs.1296 to 2238 and the per capita expenditure has also increased from Rs. 4050 to 7219. However, the growth in beneficiaries is negative (Table 3.5).

CGHS has been expanding based on certain norms. These include[3]: the criteria fixed for setting up a Central Government Health Scheme (CGHS) dispensary in a particular area are as under:

(i) <u>In an existing CGHS city</u>: For the opening of a new Allopathic CGHS dispensary in an existing CGHS city, there has to be a minimum of 2000 Card holders (serving employees of Central Government and Central Civil pensioners).

(ii) <u>Extension of CGHS to a new City:</u> For the extension of CGHS to a new city, there has to be a minimum of 6,000 Card holders.

However, due to financial and other resource constraints it is not always possible to adhere to the above criteria.

If we look further at the number of dispensaries and beneficiaries under the Central Government Health Scheme (CGHS) in India, we can also observe

Table 3.5 Total, Per Capita Expenditure and No. of Beneficiaries in CGHS (2011–2018)

Year	Total expenditure (in Crores of Rs.)	No. of beneficiaries (in Crores)	Per Capita Expenditure (in Rs.)
2010–2011	1296	0.32	4050
2011–2012	1562	0.34	4594
2012–2013	1691	0.36	4697
2013–2014	1839	0.37	4970
2014–2015	1799	0.28	6425
2015–2016	1977	0.29	6817
2016–2017	2238	0.31	7219
Growth rate	8.07	-2.35	10.66

Source: CGHS, Ministry of Health & Family Welfare.

that between 2011– 2018 there has been an increase in the number of allopathic and AYUSH dispensaries, which are growing at the rate of 0.62 and 0.64 per cent, respectively (Table 3.6). Likewise, CGHS labs and dental units have also grown at 3.01 and .01 per cent. Yet there has been a decline in the growth of beneficiaries and card holders at the rate of 2.91 and .33 per cent.

Further, the distribution of polyclinics run by CGHS in 2018 is presented in Figure 3.2 below. As could be observed there is a distribution of polyclinics which generally favours large cities such as Delhi, Chennai, Hyderabad and Nagpur, relative to other lesser sized cities in India (Figure 3.2). A similar observation could be made for distribution of AYUSH Dispensaries/ Wellness Centres in 2018 (Table 3.7).

A distribution of the total number of cards and beneficiaries is presented in Table 3.8 below. There are more than 32 lakhs of beneficiaries and 1010 lakhs of card holders in 2018 across 36 Indian cities. There are maximum and minimum beneficiaries respectively in Delhi and Gangtok (Table 3.8). A similar distribution, keeping with the number of beneficiaries, is depicted in Table 3.9. Generally, more beneficiaries and more doctors are seen in larger towns and vice-versa.

Table 3.6 CGHS Dispensaries and Beneficiaries (2001–2018)

Number of Dispensaries and Beneficiaries under Central Government Health Scheme (CGHS) in India (As on March 31, 2001 to 2018)

Years	Type of Dispensaries		Beneficiaries			
	Allopathic	AYUSH	CGHS Lab	Dental Units	Total No. of Cards	Total No. of Beneficiaries
2001	241	79	-	-	1003537	4354410
2002	244	79	-	-	1045024	4385271
2003	244	79	-	-	1041942	4457911
2004	247	86	-	-	1066251	4558794
2005	246	85	-	-	1032350	4285662
2006	244	85	-	-	911447	3301264
2007	247	85	-	-	900335	3411365
2008	247	88	-	-	857872	3209804
2009	246	86	64	21	934825	3181719
2010	246	85	67	20	847081	3152781
2011	246	85	65	22	806485	2580674
2012	250	86	67	20	1025900	3358959
2013	-	-	-	-	-	-
2014	260	90	82	21	982461	3191131
2018	287	85	73	21	1082913	3247783
Growth rate	0.64	0.62	3.01	0.01	-0.33	-2.91

Source: Ministry of Health & Family Welfare, Govt. of India. ((ON315), (ON402) & (ON832)ON1764).
Abbr.: AYUSH: Ayurveda, Yoga, Unani, Siddha, Naturopathy and Homeopathy.

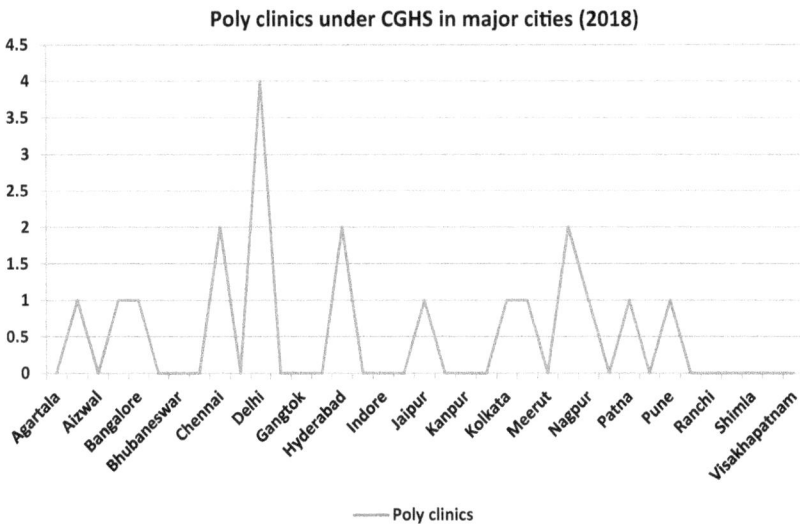

Figure 3.2 Polyclinics under CGHS in Major Cities (2018)

Source: Table 3.A.2 City-wise CGHS Dispensaries

The system of CGHS incorporates an element of public-private partnership and thus in the places where CGHS facilities are not there but beneficiaries do reside, there are empanelled clinics and Diagnostic centres (Figure 3.3). Thus across 25 cities a distribution of four types of empanelled health care facilities including hospitals, eye and dental clinics and diagnostic centres indicate respectively 558, 286, 105 and 165 empanelled established facilities (Figure 3.3). This distribution across 25 cities in regard to hospitals and diagnostic centres and eye and dental clinics is presented in Figures 3.4 and 3.5 which also suggest the norms of larger numbers of beneficiaries and more facilities prorate.

Despite a fair distribution of these CGHS facilities, the performance of CGHS has not always been satisfactory. A number of issues from time to time have been raised by many studies. For instance, mid-term appraisal of the Tenth Five-Year Plan (2002–2007) had observed "low satisfaction levels with CGHS which related to poor emergency services, non-availability of medicines, and inconvenient timings." (GoI, 2008). Similarly in 2013, another report presented to Parliament on the functioning of CGHS scheme also raised a number of issues including scarcity of doctors due to lack of timely recruitments, timings of CGHS services, infrastructure and behavioural issues (GoI, 2013). There have been complaints about long waiting periods, inadequate supply of medicines and equipment and unhygienic conditions (Devdasan, 2006). Using four indicators of patient satisfaction, namely accessibility, environment and

Table 3.7 Distribution of AYUSH Dispensaries/Wellness Centres (2018)

*Selected State/City-wise Number of Allopathic, Ayurveda, Yoga, Unani, Siddha
and Homeopathy (AYUSH) Dispensaries/Wellness Centres under Central
Government Health Scheme (CGHS) in India
(As on 10.08.2018)*

States/UTs	City	Allopathic	Ayurvedic	Homeopathic	Unaani	Sidha	Yoga
Andhra Pradesh	Visakhapatnam	1	0	0	0	0	0
Assam	Guwahati	5	0	1	0	0	0
Bihar	Patna	5	1	1	0	0	0
Chandigarh	Chandigarh	1	0	0	0	0	0
Chhattisgarh	Raipur	1	0	0	0	0	0
Delhi	Delhi	86	12	13	5	1	4
Goa	Panaji	1	0	0	0	0	0
Gujarat	Ahmedabad	8	1	1	1	0	0
	Gandhinagar	1	0	0	0	0	0
Haryana	Faridabad	1	0	0	0	0	0
	Gurgaon	2	1	0	0	0	0
Himachal Pradesh	Shimla	1	0	0	0	0	0
Jammu and Kashmir	Jammu	2	0	0	0	0	0
Jharkhand	Ranchi	3	0	0	0	0	0
Karnataka	Bengaluru	10	2	1	1	0	0
Kerala	Thiruvananthapuram	3	1	1	0	0	0
Madhya Pradesh	Bhopal	2	0	0	0	0	0
	Jabalpur	5	0	0	0	0	0
	Indore	1	0	0	0	0	0
Maharashtra	Mumbai	26	2	3	0	0	0
	Nagpur	11	2	1	0	0	0
	Pune	9	1	2	0	0	0
Manipur	Imphal	1	0	0	0	0	0
Meghalaya	Shillong	2	0	0	0	0	0
Mizoram	Aizawl	1	0	0	0	0	0
Nagaland	Kohima	1	0	0	0	0	0
Odisha	Bhubaneshwar	3	1	0	0	0	0
Puducherry	Puducherry	1	0	0	0	0	0
Rajasthan	Jaipur	7	1	1	0	0	0
Sikkim	Gangtok	1	0	0	0	0	0
Tamil Nadu	Chennai	14	1	1	0	2	0
Telangana	Hyderabad	13	2	2	2	0	0
Tripura	Agartala	1	0	0	0	0	0
Uttar Pradesh	Allahabad	7	1	1	0	0	0
	Ghaziabad	1	0	0	0	0	0
	Greater Noida	1	0	0	0	0	0
	Indirapuram	1	0	0	0	0	0
	Kanpur	9	1	2	0	0	0
	Lucknow	9	1	1	1	0	0
	Noida	2	0	0	0	0	0
	Meerut	6	1	1	0	0	0
	Sahibabad	1	0	0	0	0	0
Uttarakhand	Dehradun	2	0	0	0	0	0
West Bengal	Kolkata	18	1	2	1	0	0
India		287	33	35	10	3	4

Source: Lok Sabha Unstarred Question No. 4092, dated on 10.08.2018.

Table 3.8 Distribution of Cards and Beneficiaries under CGHS (2018)

Selected City-wise Number of Cards and Beneficiaries under
Central Government Health Scheme (CGHS) in India
(As on 13.02.2018)

City	Total no. of cards	Total no. of beneficiaries
Agartala	518	1612
Ahmedabad	15701	45807
Allahabad	18443	59260
Bangalore	41044	116170
Bhopal	5589	15208
Bhubaneswar	6447	19744
Chandigarh	12759	31249
Chennai	41891	111706
Dehradun	10423	24888
Delhi	490088	1601099
Gandhinagar	2559	9532
Gangtok	4	8
Goa	60	203
Guwahati	13560	46303
Hyderabad	65867	184799
Imphal	147	590
Indore	628	1387
Jabalpur	35138	84780
Jaipur	18617	54950
Jammu	1108	2716
Kanpur	30919	83787
Kohima	50	147
Kolkata	56530	147750
Lucknow	21421	68788
Meerut	13914	41105
Mumbai	56702	171059
Nagpur	30019	79366
Patna	13040	42843
Puducherry	508	1611
Pune	48254	114098
Raipur	35	72
Ranchi	4881	15451
Shillong	5102	17660
Shimla	803	2076
Thiruvananthapuram	15345	38082
Visakhapatnam	4799	11877
India	1082913	3247783

Source: Ministry of Health & Family Welfare, Govt. of India. (ON1764).

Table 3.9 Distribution of Doctors under CGHS in Major Cities (2018)

City-wise Number of Doctors Working in Central Government
Health Scheme (CGHS) Dispensaries in India
(As on June 30, 2018)

City	Total no. of doctors working
Agartala	1
Ahmedabad + Gandhi	16
Aizawl	1
Allahabad	18
Bangalore	54
Bhopal + Indore	6
Bhubaneshwar	8
Chandigarh	7
Chennai + Puducherry	58
Dehradun	7
Delhi	853
Gangtok	1
Guwahati	9
Hyderabad + Visakhapatnam	96
Imphal	1
Jabalpur	7
Jaipur	39
Jammu	2
Kanpur	33
Kohima	1
Kolkata	84
Lucknow	49
Meerut	23
Mumbai	89
Nagpur	45
Panaji	1
Patna	29
Pune	45
Raipur	1
Ranchi	9
Shillong	4
Shimla	2
Trivandrum	13
Total	1612

Source: Lok Sabha Unstarred Question No. 665, dated on 20.07.2018.

the behaviour of doctors and other staff, Vellakkal, Juyal, and Mehdi (2010) have reported lowest levels (0.48) among CGHS beneficiaries in comparison to the Ex-Servicemen Contributory Health Scheme. Studies on CGHS dispensaries in Kolkata also found varying levels of patient satisfaction, 60 per

Number of Hospitals, Eye clinics, dental clinics and diagnostic
centres empanelled under CGHS across 25 cities in India (2015)

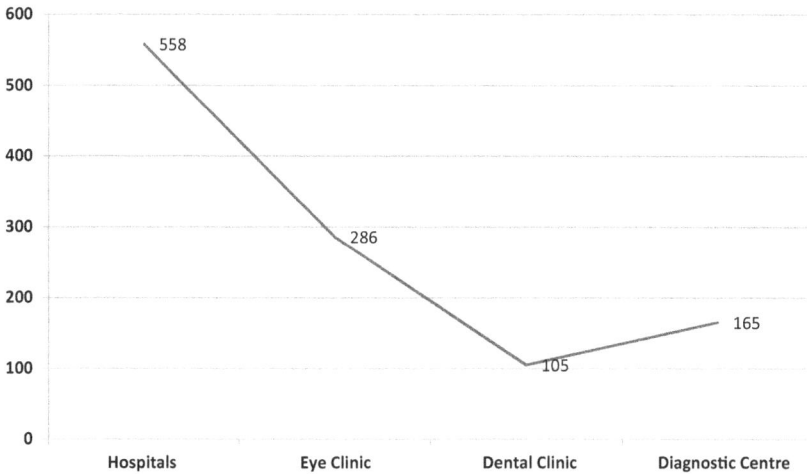

Figure 3.3 Empanelled Clinics and Diagnostic Centres under CGHS (2015).
Source: https://cghs.nic.in

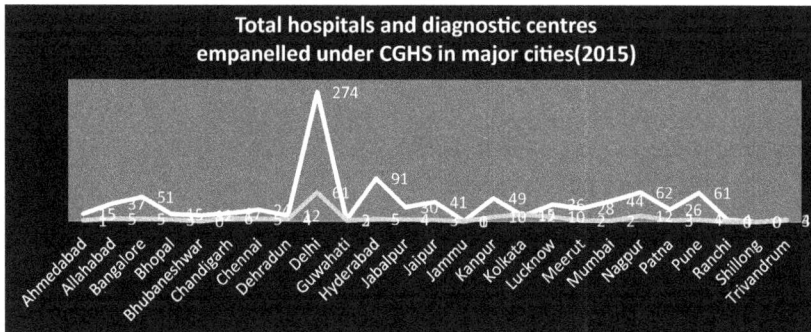

Figure 3.4 Total Hospitals and Diagnostic Centres Empanelled under CGHS (2015).
Source: https://cghs.nic.in

cent in 2002–2003 and 65 per cent in 2008–2009 (Chattopadhyay et al., 2013). Satisfaction levels were lower among the pensioner's dependants and those with lower incomes, suggesting differential treatment based on influence and power of the patient. The gaps identified were an absence of CGHS hospitals with inpatient facilities, drug supply issues and long waiting times, inadequate health personnel and poor infrastructure facilities such as toilet,

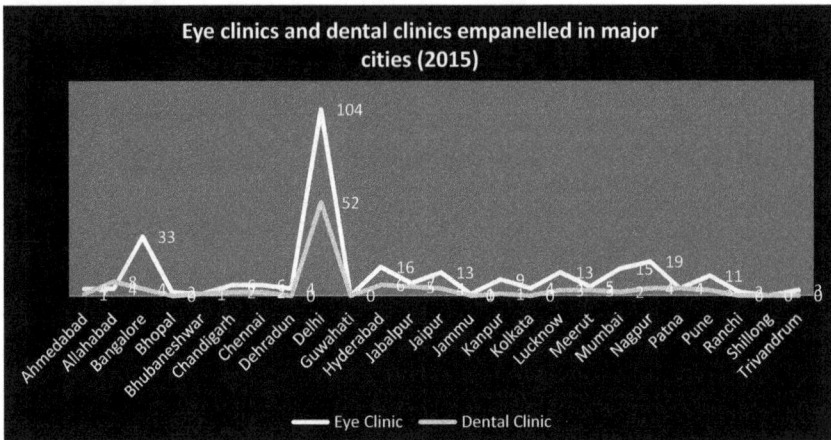

Figure 3.5 Eye and Dental Clinics Empanelled under CGHS (2015).

Source: https://cghs.nic.in

drinking water, sitting arrangements, overcrowding and laboratory services (Haldar et al., 2008). Short service hours and a lack of infrastructure prevent the possibility of providing round the clock emergency care. The needs of patients included ambulance facility, immunisation services, own inpatient hospital, specialists and services in Indian systems of medicine. Other service issues include long waiting times, inadequate medicines, equipment and staff, and often unhygienic conditions (Gumber, 2002).

Another study by Kumari, Tripathy and Bhaskar (2016), attempts to evaluate the working of the Central Government Health Scheme (CGHS) by assessing beneficiaries' satisfaction. The study is based on a primary survey of 412 CGHS beneficiaries across six cities in the country. These include Ranchi, Kolkata, Patna, Jaipur, Shillong, and Allahabad. The survey revealed that the patients are reasonably satisfied with the health care services of both empanelled private health care providers and the dispensaries/polyclinics under the CGHS. They also observed that respondents are relatively more satisfied with the former than the latter. The CGHS empanelled private health care providers are dissatisfied with the terms and conditions of empanelment, especially the low tariffs for their services as compared to prevailing market rates of respective cities and the delays in reimbursements from the schemes. This study suggests enhancing the quality of health care in the dispensaries/polyclinics of the CGHS and steps for sustainable public-private partnership.

Nonetheless CGHS beneficiaries have much to be satisfied about the scheme. Enrolment in service areas is compulsory and contribution means-based thereby enabling risk pooling. The coverage is comprehensive, without any financial ceiling. It offers referral to private facilities of choice, and access to a wide range of prescription medicines (Sarwal, 2015).

Employees' State Insurance Scheme (ESIS)

The Employees' State Insurance Act, 1948 envisaged an integrated need-based social insurance scheme that would protect the interests of workers in contingencies such as sickness, maternity, temporary or permanent physical disablement, death due to employment and injury resulting in loss of wages or earning capacity. The Act also guarantees medical care to workers and their immediate dependents. ESIS is a contributory scheme on the patterns of social health insurance. The existing wage limit for coverage under the Act is Rs. 15,000/- per month (w.e.f. 01/05/2010). The scheme is being implemented in all states except Manipur, Sikkim, Arunachal Pradesh and Mizoram. It is also being implemented in Delhi and Chandigarh.

Medical benefit is one part of the benefits under ESIS, but the scheme also includes other benefits for sickness, maternity, disablement etc. Full medical care is provided to an insured person and his family members from the day he enters insurable employment. There is no ceiling on expenditure on the treatment of an insured person or his family member, and treatment can be availed at primary, secondary and tertiary levels. Medical care is also provided to retired and permanently disabled insured persons and their spouses on payment of a token annual premium of Rs.120/-.

Under the ESI scheme, employees contribute 1.75 per cent of their wages and the employers contribute 4.75 per cent of the wages of eligible beneficiaries/employees towards premium payments. Employees earning less than Rs. 50 per day are exempted from contribution towards premium payments. The contributions made by the employees and the employers are deposited in a common pool known as the ESI Fund, which is used for meeting administrative expenses as well as cash and medical benefits to insured persons (IP) and their dependents. The state governments, as per the ESI Act, contribute 12.5 per cent of the total expenditure (within the per capita ceiling of Rs.1000 per annum) incurred by the ESIC on medical care in respective states. The objectives of ESIS are to provide benefits in cash and kind which include: Medical Benefit (for self and family); Sickness Benefit (for self); Maternity Benefit (for self); Disablement Benefit, both temporary and permanent (for self); dependents' benefit (for family); Funeral Expenses (to a person who performs the last rites of an IP); rehabilitation allowance (for self); vocational rehabilitation for the IPs; Old age Medicare (for self and spouse); and medical bonus (for insured women and IP's wife)[4].

The following Table indicates the coverage situation. The ESIS covers a very large population of workers which are more than 12 crores, and 3.19 crore families benefit from this (Table 3.10).

However, total expenditure on medical benefit under ESIS has been growing at a higher rate relative to either of number of beneficiaries or per capita expenditure on medical benefit between 2009 and 2017 (Table 3.11, last row).

Financially over the years from 2001–2013, the scheme has been running in a sound position with the growth of income being higher than expenditure (Table 3.12).

Across 26 states and union territories, there is a considerable variation in terms of number of IPs, per capita care on normal and super speciality care (Table 3.13, columns 3, 6, 8 and 10). In 2009–2010 for instance, in regard to mean IPS, maximum were in Maharashtra and max per capita expenditure was in Delhi (Table 3.13, third from last row). Likewise minimum for these in the same parameters were Tripura and Uttarakhand respectively (Table 3.13, second from last row).

However, in terms of income from contributions, the maximum and minimum was shown respectively for Maharashtra and Assam in 2009–2010 (Table 3.14). Even within a state there are considerable variations across different towns (see Table 3.A.6 Selected State-wise Cash and Other Benefits under ESIS and Table 3.A.7 Selected State-wise Other Benefits given under ESIS).

Some of the studies which have looked into ESIS functioning indicate both a satisfactory as well as unsatisfactory performance. For instance, an all India level study by Ahmad (2001) indicates that the ESIC has progressively expanded the series of benefits to the workers and also achieved a gradual

Table 3.10 Coverage of ESIS (as on March 31, 2017)

No. of insured person family units	3.19 crore
No. of employees covered	2.93 crore
Total no. of beneficiaries	12.4 crore

Source: Employee State Insurance Corporation.

Table 3.11 Trends in Coverage, Income and Expenditure on ESIS

Year	Expenditure on medical benefit (In Rs. crore)	No. of beneficiaries (in crores)	Per capita expenditure on medical benefit (Rs)
2009	1272.83	5.02	254
2010	1778.61	5.55	320
2011	2306.83	6.03	383
2012	2858.87	6.64	431
2013	4058.13	7.21	563
2014	4859.9	7.58	641
2015	5714.34	7.89	724
2016	6112.97	8.28	738
2017	6256.57	12.4	505
growth rate	22.99	9.58	12.24

Source: Employee State Insurance Corporation.

Table 3.12 Income and Expenditure of Employees State Insurance Corporation (ESIC) in India (Growth 2001–2013)

Years	Total income	Total expenditure
2001	156,254	101,980.9
2002	172,878	104162.5
2003	169,922	105,319.8
2004	197,192	117,047.5
2005	224,606	125,819.5
2006	241,062	127,896.2
2007	310,811	134,864.4
2008	398,932	154,885.8
2009	445,246	206,883
2010	508,518	271,180.3
2012	837,355	419,099.6
2013	1E+06	564,757.8
growth rate	18.48	15.62

Source: Table 3.A.5 Income and Expenditure of Employees State Insurance Corporation (ESIC) in India (2001–2007, as on 31st March).

increasing trend in all its fields of operation. The study covers the whole of the country from 1970 to 1998. It reveals that the ESIS Corporation has been playing a dominant role in creating a welfare state in the country with the ultimate goal of socio-economic advancement. Thus, the net impact on of this social security in India has maintained comprehension, integration, absolution of employers' liabilities, industrial improvement, standard of living and improvement in economic and managerial benefits.

However, another study at state level, focussing on Kerala by Jose (2006) indicates; a) that most of the insured persons in factories and establishments are not fully aware of the ESI benefits. Compared to the insured persons, the employers are better informed about the ESI benefits. The Corporation is not keen on giving adequate information on the ESI Scheme to the insured persons and employers. The insured persons are not satisfied with the measures taken by the Corporation for providing information on the ESI Scheme; b) all insured persons do not prefer ESI dispensaries for the treatment. Lack of doctors, lack of medicines and other facilities for treatment and lack of confidence are the factors preventing them from taking treatment from ESI dispensaries. The insured persons who are taking treatment from ESI dispensaries are not satisfied with the various services/facilities provided in ESI dispensaries for treatment; c) all the insured persons referred to ESI hospitals are not taking further treatments from ESI hospitals due to factors such as the lack of doctors and medicines. Other facilities for treatment and travel difficulties prevent some insured persons from taking further treatments from ESI hospitals. The insured persons who are taking further treatment from ESI hospitals are not satisfied with the various services/facilities provided in ESI hospitals for treatment; d) the amount of cash benefit given by the

Table 3.13 State-wise Expenditure Incurred on Provision of Medical Care under Employees State Insurance Corporation (ESIC) in India (2009–2010)

States/UTs	Approved No. of IPs as on 31.03.2009	31.03.2010	Mean	Expen-diture incurred by state/UTs (in lacs)	Per capita expenditure incurred by State/UTs (in Rs.)	Expenditure on model/ESIC hospital (in lacs)	Expenditure on super speciality (in lacs)	Total expenditure (in lacs)	Total per capita expenditure (in Rs.)
Andhra Pradesh	889,217	1,012,800	951,009	15,604.05	1640.79	2262.43	2310.62	20,177.1	2121.65
Assam	54,855	58,870	56,863	778.96	1369.9	893.04	3.68	1675.68	2946.9
Bihar	72,258	90,300	81,279	708.27	871.41	725.98	130	1564.25	1924.54
Chandigarh (Adm.)	72,743	69,450	71,097	493.47	694.08	1070.72	0.4	1564.59	2200.66
Chhattisgarh	109,988	193,050	151,519	647.07	427.06	0	70	717.07	473.25
Delhi	820,180	906,500	863,340	21,370.41	2475.32	6217.38	3909.97	31,497.76	3648.36
Gujarat	719,082	752,950	736,016	10,107.39	1373.26	2179.12	741	13,027.51	1770
Goa	146,256	129,150	137,703	1176.94	854.69	0	25	1201.94	272.85
Haryana	741,552	889,900	815,726	7488.24	917.98	0	570.73	8058.97	987.95
Himachal Pradesh	148,123	173700	160912	611.5	380.02	0	10.12	621.62	386.31
Jammu and Kashmir	62,718	78800	70759	256.15	362	320.46	30	606.61	857.29
Jharkhand	153,199	176200	164700	1244.72	755.75	910.92	59	2214.64	1344.65
Karnataka	1,493,581	1554100	1523841	9026.87	592.38	5085.75	1913.7	16026.32	1051.71
Kerala	597,540	622650	610095	6655.4	1090.88	2314	970.95	9940.35	1629.31
Madhya Pradesh	289,526	296300	292913	4880.34	1666.14	2368.41	43.25	7292	2489.48
Maharashtra	1,784,993	1802700	1799847	9235.39	514.84	3487.44	576.71	13299.54	741.4
Meghalaya	5332	6190	5761	96.95	1682.87	0	2.77	99.72	1730.95
Orissa	189,866	236500	213183	2283.07	1070.94	365.22	108.98	2757.27	1293.38
Puducherry	90,566	105600	98083	1067.11	1087.97	0	62.9	1130.01	1152.1
Punjab	616,495	697950	657223	5009.41	762.21	1718.78	381.77	7109.96	1081.82
Rajasthan	516,001	534550	525276	4953.7	943.07	1604.34	177.53	6735.57	1282.29
Tamil Nadu	1,583,470	1827800	1705635	13043.05	764.7	3421.1	268.26	16732.41	981.01
Uttar Pradesh	823,827	860550	842189	8554.71	1015.77	3719.73	364.82	12639.26	1500.76
Uttarakhand	175,172	233500	204336	379.69	185.82	0	22	401.69	196.58
West Bengal	780,577	988100	884339	17706.88	2002.27	3293.52	836.04	21836.44	2469.24
Tripura	460	1840	1150	37.49	3260	0	0	37.49	3260
max	1,784,993	1,827,800	1,793,847	21,370.41	3260	6217.38	3909.97	31,497.76	3648.36
min	460	1840	1150	37.49	185.82	0	0	37.49	196.58
India	12,937,577	14,300,000	13,618,789	143,417.2	-	41,958.34	13590.2	198,965.8	1460.97

Source: Employees' State Insurance Corporation. (12651)

Table 3.14 State-wise Contributions under ESIS

Selected State-wise Contribution Income under Employees State Insurance (ESI) Scheme in India (2009–2010)

States/UTs	Income (Rs. in Lakh)
Andhra Pradesh	29,190.38
Assam	1206.79
Bihar	1541.04
Delhi	26,601.22
West Bengal	26,405.79
Haryana	27,998.31
Karnataka	43,152.88
Madhya Pradesh	6934.44
Chhattisgarh	2222.21
Punjab	14,414.95
Chandigarh	2654.4
Jharkhand	3307.71
Goa	3220.63
Maharashtra	69,664.08
Tamil Nadu	52,182.38
Pondicherry	2406.28
Rajasthan	11,318.31
Gujrat	16,678.9
Orissa	4301.95
Jammu & Kashmir	1355.41
Himachal Pradesh	3549.66
Uttar Pradesh	20,103.17
Kerala	14,212.66
Uttarakhand	4976.64
India	389,600.19

Source: Lok Sabha Unstarred Question No. 1306, dated on 02.08.2010.

Corporation is insufficient, and there is delay in getting the payment of cash benefits apart from the sickness and other benefits; e) respondents are satisfied with the services of the staff for claiming the cash benefits except the sickness benefit. The advisory bodies of the ESI Corporation are not satisfactory. This is owing to infrequent meetings, no timely constitution of the Regional Boards and the Local Committees and no adequate representation of the employees and employers in the various advisory boards of the Corporation except the Local Committees. However, the study expressed a satisfactory fund management by ESIS.

Another state-level study focussing on Tamil Nadu also pointed out some of the inadequacies in performance of ESIS (Dash and Muraleedharan, 2011). It carried out a survey of about 900 beneficiaries in the Chennai region from August 2007 to March 2008. The beneficiaries were chosen from four different sectors: textiles, engineering, food and beverages (restaurants in particular) and leather and leather products. It tried to assess the utilisation pattern of the ESI facilities and the extent that the ESI Scheme helps to protect the beneficiaries from the catastrophic health expenditure. The findings show that the overall utilisation level is very low due to perceived low-quality drugs, long waiting periods, insolence of personnel, long waiting spells to unusual delays in reimbursement of money spent on treatment outside, lack of or low interest of employers and low awareness of ESI procedures. The study suggests that the government could improve access to health care by constructing more Scheme facilities or adding more private facilities to the panel of recognised hospitals where beneficiaries can get treatment. The basic infrastructure of the existing facilities could be improved to provide a higher quality of service by increasing availability of basic diagnostic equipment available, nursing personnel, laboratory services and better sanitary conditions. Also, the study suggests the introduction of a multiple card system for better utilisation with the choice of the convenient locations of beneficiaries.

Rashtriya Swasthya Bima Yojana (RSBY)

Rashtriya Swasthya Bima Yojana (RSBY, "National Health Insurance Programme"), is a government-run health insurance programme. It is aimed at covering people below the poverty line (BPL). It provides health insurance coverage to the unrecognised sector workers belonging to the BPL category and their family members. It provides for cashless insurance for hospitalisation and treatment in public and private hospitals. The scheme began enrolment on April 1, 2008, and has been implemented in 25 states of India. By 2016, a total of 36 million families had been enrolled (Table 3.A.8 Families Enrolled under RSBY (2012–17, States and All India)). For most of the states, the number of BPL families enrolled has fallen short of targets (Figure 3.6).

According to Tendulkar, the committee estimates about 37.2 per cent of the total Indian population are BPL, but RSBY had enrolled only around 10 per cent of the Indian population by March 31, 2011. It is expected to cost the exchequer at least ₹3,350 crore (US$480 million) a year to cover the entire BPL population

RSBY scheme collects Rs. 30 from every "below poverty line" (BPL) family holding a yellow ration card. This is a registration fee to get a biometric-enabled smart card containing their fingerprints and photographs. Using this smart card, enrolled families can receive inpatient medical care of up to Rs. 30,000 (US$430) per family per year in any of the empanelled hospitals. The scheme also covers pre-existing illnesses from day one, for the head of the household, spouses and up to three dependent children or parents.

In the Union Budget, the government made a total allocation of Rs. 5133 crores towards RSBY (Table 3.15).

Gap between targets and enrolled BPL in RSBY

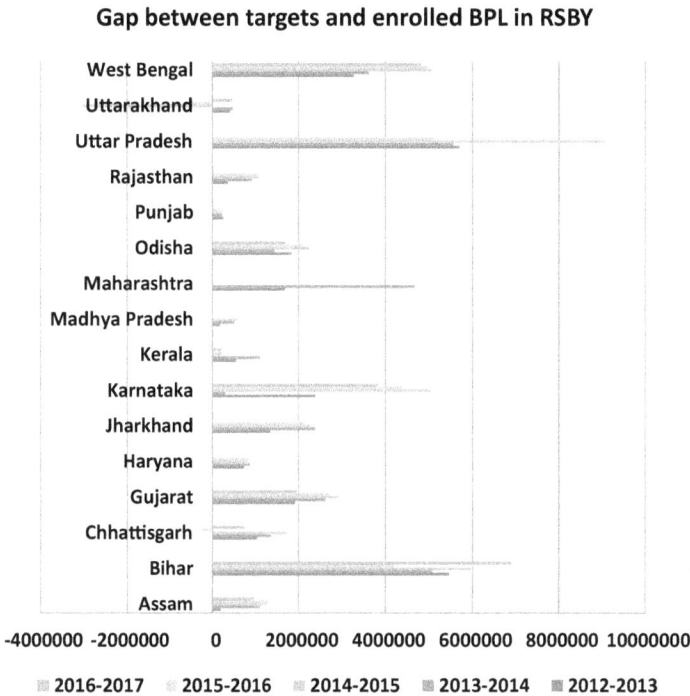

Figure 3.6 Shortfall between targets and achievements in enrolment of RSBY in major states (2012–2017). Source: Table 3.A.8 Families Enrolled under RSBY (2012–17, States and All India).

The scheme was appreciated by the World Bank, the UN and the ILO as one of the world's best health insurance schemes. Though Germany, which has a social security system of insurance which is voucher based, had shown interest in the smart card-based model. One of the big changes that this scheme entails is bringing investments to unserved areas. Most private investments in health care in India are in tertiary or specialised care in urban areas. However, with RSBY, companies like Global Healthcare Systems, a company based out of Kolkata and funded by Tier I Capital Funds like Sequoia Capital and Elevar Equity are setting up state-of–the-art hospitals in semi urban-rural settings (The Economic Times. 3 February 2012).

RSBY is a government sponsored scheme for the BPL population of India. The majority of the financing, about 75 per cent, is provided by the Government of India (GOI), while the remainder is paid by the respective state government. Government of India's contribution is 90 per cent in the case of north-eastern states and Jammu and Kashmir and respective state governments need to pay only 10 per cent of the premium. RSBY involves a

Table 3.15 Budget Allocation for RSBY (2007–2017)

Budget Allocation for Expansion of Rashtriya
Swasthya Bima Yojana (RSBY) in India
(2007–2008 to 2016–2017) (Rs. in Crore)

Years	Budget	Revised	Final	Expenditure
	Estimates	Estimates	Estimates	
2007–08	5.00	5.00	5.00	-
2008–09	251.00	251.00	251.00	103.00
2009–10	350.00	350.00	350.00	265.00
2010–11	350.00	548.00	548.00	512.00
2011–12	313.42	984.30	984.30	926.00
2012–13	1568.56	1177.60	1177.60	1002.00
2013–14	1265.00	847.00	891.92	888.00
2014–15	1319.30	539.74	-	551.00
2015–16	700.00	-	-	449.00
2016–17	-	-	-	437.00
Total	6122.28	4702.64	4207.82	5133.00

Source: Health Family Welfare, Govt. of India. (ON1764);loksabha Unstarred Question No.1526, dated on 21.07.2014;Lok Sabha Unstarred Question No.1146, dated on 02.03.2015;Lok Sabha Unstarred Question No.2152, dated on 11.12.2015

set of complex and inter-related activities. Beneficiaries need to pay only Rs. 30 as the registration fee. This amount is used for incurring administrative expenses under the scheme.

State governments engage in a competitive public bidding process and select a public or private insurance company licensed to provide health insurance by the Insurance Regulatory Development Authority (IRDA) or enabled by a central legislation. The technical bids with the lowest financial bid are then selected for providing health insurance in the state. The insurer thus agrees to cover the benefit package prescribed by GOI through a cashless facility and the use of smart cards.

Each contract is specified on the basis of an individual district in a state and the insurer agrees to set up an office in each district. While more than one insurer can operate in a particular state, only one insurer can operate in a single district at any given point in time.

State government must prepare and submit the BPL data in an electronic format specified by Government of India. The format requires details of all family members including name, father or husband's name for the head of household, age, gender and relationship with the head of household. Respective state governments need to convert their existing BPL data to this format for each district and send this data to Government of India, which in turn checks the compatibility of this data with the standard format. However, state governments alone are responsible for the accuracy of their BPL lists.

Preparation of BPL data in the specified format is necessary for implementing the scheme in the state.

Thus, an electronic list of eligible BPL households is provided to the insurer using a pre-specified data format. An enrolment schedule for each village, along with dates, is prepared by the insurance company with the help of the district level officials. As per the schedule, the BPL list is posted in each village at enrolment stations and prominent places prior to the enrolment, and the date and location of the enrolment in the village is publicised in advance. Mobile enrolment stations are set up at local centres (e.g., public schools) in each village. These stations are equipped by the insurer with the hardware required to collect biometric information (fingerprints) and photographs of the members of the household covered and a printer to print smart cards with a photo. The smart card, along with an information pamphlet describing the scheme and the list of hospitals, is provided on the spot once the beneficiary has paid the 30-rupee fee. The process normally takes less than ten minutes. The cards are handed over in a plastic cover.[5]

Once the insurance company is selected, it has to empanel both public and private health care providers in the project and nearby districts. The empanelment of the hospitals is done based on prescribed criteria. The insurer may empanel enough hospitals in the district so that beneficiaries need not travel very far to access the health care services. For empanelment of the public hospitals, the insurer needs to coordinate with the respective health department of the state.

Each of the empanelled hospitals should install necessary hardware and software so that smart card transactions can be processed. They should also set up a special RSBY desk with trained staff. The hospital list should allow for both public and private hospitals who agree to participate. The insurer must also provide a list of RSBY empanelled hospitals to the beneficiaries at the time of enrolment. This list can be revised at periodic intervals as more and more hospitals are added in the list. When empanelment takes place, a nationally unique hospital ID number is generated so that transactions can be tracked at each stage.[6]

After rendering the service to the patient, the hospitals need to send an electronic report to the insurer/Third Party Administrator (TPA). The Insurer/TPA, after going through the records information, will make the payment to the hospital within a specified time period which has been agreed between the Insurer and the hospital.

With the smart card, and consequent to the commencement of the policy, the beneficiary shall be able to use health service facilities in any of the RSBY empanelled hospital across India. Any hospital which is empanelled under RSBY by any insurance company will provide cashless treatment to the beneficiary[7].

There is a considerable increase in overall empanelled hospitals, both in public and private sectors, who are providing care to RSBY smart card holders. In 2016–2017, for instance, all India empanelled public and private hospitals numbered 3771 and 4926, respectively (Table 3.16). Among some of the major states, maximum empanelment was depicted for Gujarat both in private and public sector hospitals with the number of empanelled hospitals in the state as 1251 and 638 respectively (Table 3.16, row 5).

The number of smart cards issued under RSBY also increased at the all-India level from nearly 39 lakhs to around 3.4 crores between 2008–2010 and 2012–2013 (Table 3.17, last row). Among the major states the maximum number of smart cards were issued in Uttar Pradesh in 2008–2009 (Table 3.17, 4th row from below) and the numbers remained as 834,871. However, in 2012–2013 this figure, at 6,762,779. was highest for Bihar (Table 3.17, row3).

In terms of hospitalisation benefit availed under RSBY, there has been a steady increase at the all-India level, and the respective numbers of hospitalisation between 2008–2009 and 2016–2017 increased from 12,541 to 2,205,598 (Table 3.18, last row). Among the major states the maximum number of hospitalisations respectively in 2008–2009 and 2016–2017 were depicted for Gujarat at 3,286 (in 2008–2009) and Chhattisgarh at 729,562 (in 2016–2017) (Table 3.18, rows 8 and 6 respectively).

However, a comparison with both the number of smart card holders and hospitalisations in the latest year of 2012–2013 indicates Kerala as the highest user at percentage of numbers of hospitalisation to number of smart card holders at 24.5 per cent (Figure 3.7).

Overall, there has been a steady increase in the total number of beneficiaries under RSBY between 2008 and 2014, with the respective numbers

Table 3.16 Selected State-wise Hospitals Empanelment under RSBY (2016–2017)

Selected State-wise Number of Hospitals (Private and Public) Empanelled under Rashtriya Swasthya Bima Yojana (RSBY) Scheme in India (2016–2017)

States	No. of private hospitals	No. of public hospitals
Assam	47	141
Bihar	1001	151
Chhattisgarh	640	395
Gujarat	1251	638
Karnataka	541	653
Kerala	271	278
Odisha	211	424
Uttarakhand	66	94
West Bengal	822	481
India	4926	3771

Source: Lok Sabha Unstarred Question No. 3399, dated on 04.08.2017.

Table 3.17 Selected State-wise Number of Smart Cards Issued under Rashtriya Swasthya Bima Yojana (RSBY) in India (2008–2009 to 2012–2013 and 2016–2017)

States/UTs	Smart Cards Issued				
	2008–09	2009–10	2010–11	2011–12	2012–13
Andhra Pradesh	0	0	0	0	1408
Assam	-	81,565	204,465	204,548	174,968
Bihar	557,002	2,038,909	5,101,901	7,184,460	6,762,779
Chhattisgarh	0	927,672	1,230,378	1,384,680	1,678,971
Goa	1679	3505	0	0	0
Gujarat	670,517	682,354	1,919,086	1,826,204	1,810,326
Haryana	401,587	682,354	621,741	584,683	388,587
Jharkhand	101,219	434,762	1,329,254	1,167,456	1,258,010
Karnataka	-	36,971	157,405	893,069	1,680,913
Kerala	703,570	1,173,388	1,796,315	1,748,471	2,743,665
Madhya Pradesh	0	0	0	0	101,476
Maharashtra	135,804	1,440,407	1,516,687	2,178,037	2,263,854
Odisha	-	341,653	433,079	1,287,463	3,392,551
Punjab	76,528	169306	193,541	220,486	212,371
Rajasthan	120,123	*	*	0	732,778
Tamil Nadu	57,925	149,520	0	0	0
Uttar Pradesh	83,4871	4,296,865	4,233,626	4,145,925	4,674,997
Uttarakhand	50,071	53,940	335,424	338,879	305,917
West Bengal	119,327	802,974	3,527,137	4,490,145	4,856,475
India	3,961,855	13,865,338	23,362,463	28,570,697	34,415,913

Source: Same as Table 3.16.

increasing from 12,541 to 1,676,334 (Table 3.19, last row). Among the states which continue with RSBY in 2014–2015, the maximum number of beneficiaries among the major states were at 329,631 in West Bengal (Table 3.19, 2nd Row from below).

A further look at the workers in unorganised sectors utilising RSBY suggests that these numbers increased from (Table 3.20, last row nearly 3.8 crores to 4.1 crores between 2013–2016 at the all-India level. At the state level, maximum workers under unorganised sectors with RSBY were in Bihar at 6,102,774 and 6,888,208 respectively in 2013–2014 and 2015–2016 (Table 3.20, row 5).

Some of the studies carried out to analyse the overall functioning of RSBY have indicated both positive and negative features of the scheme. For instance, a study by the Council for Social Development (2014),[8] has concluded that the government-financed health insurance scheme had little or no impact on medical impoverishment in India.

In fact, the study found that despite high enrolment in RSBY, catastrophic health expenditures (when medical expenses push a family into poverty),

Table 3.18 Persons Hospitalised under Rashtriya Swasthya Bima Yojana (RSBY) in India (2008–2009 to 2012–2013 and 2016–2017)

States/UTs	Number of Persons Hospitalised					
	2008–09	2009–10	2010–11	2011–12	2012–13	2016–17
Andhra Pradesh	0	0	0	0	0	-
Assam	-	-	7224	13,253	6717	25,677
Bihar	69	16,660	98,570	209,191	164,043	84,417
Chhattisgarh	0	26	41,819	142,182	144,704	729,562
Goa	0	2	0	0	0	-
Gujarat	3286	45,273	50,402	82,328	112,138	55,577
Haryana	3220	35,890	40,395	46,396	24,732	-
Jharkhand	305	7782	35,061	26,303	37,843	-
Karnataka	149	40,167	1999	2528	32,185	65,679
Kerala	149	40167	380,422	694,676	671,743	387,344
Madhya Pradesh	0	0	0	0	656	-
Maharashtra	4	6632	30,887	64,292	47,459	-
Odisha	-	-	3792	8615	136,368	212,568
Punjab	161	1685	8317	9075	8051	-
Rajasthan	664	-	0	0	2328	-
Tamil Nadu	-	221	1475	0	0	-
Uttar Pradesh	-	28,739	360,144	216,927	86,455	-
Uttarakhand	140	64	3522	18,300	4709	54
West Bengal	-	2347	33,054	152,626	20,667	524,931
India	12,541	188,983	1,175,456	1,746,980	1,775,610	2205598

*: Rajasthan Government has discontinued the scheme; the states Goa and Tamil Nadu have discontinued the scheme

Source: Lok Sabha Unstarred Question No. 2754, dated on 7.12.2009,
Lok Sabha Unstarred Question No. 207, dated on 26.07.2010,
Rajya Sabha Unstarred Question No. 2674, dated on 18.08.2010,
Lok Sabha Unstarred Question No. 3106, dated on 29.11.2010,
Lok Sabha Starred Question No. 158, dated on 07.03.2011,
Rajya Sabha Unstarred Question No. 1828, dated on 17.08.2011,
Lok Sabha Unstarred Question No. 2781, dated on 12.12.2011,
Lok Sabha Unstarred Question No. 2358, dated on 27.08.2012,
Lok Sabha Unstarred Question No. 1967, dated on 26.03.2012,
Lok Sabha Unstarred Question No. 4478, dated on 22.04.2013 &
Lok Sabha Unstarred Question No. 3399, dated on 04.08.2014.

hospitalisation expenditure and the percentage of total household outgo on out-of-pocket (OOP) expenses – medicines and other consumables that are not reimbursed by insurance – have steadily increased, for both in-patients and outpatients, over the last two decades. It compared data before and after the launch of RSBY to understand the emerging trends in out-of-pocket expenditure for medical care. This was to analyse the impact of RSBY and its financial risk protection to beneficiaries. "Between 2004-05 and 2011-12, hospitalisation expenses have increased at a much higher rate (9.2%)

Percentage of smart card hospitalised in 2012-13 under RSBY

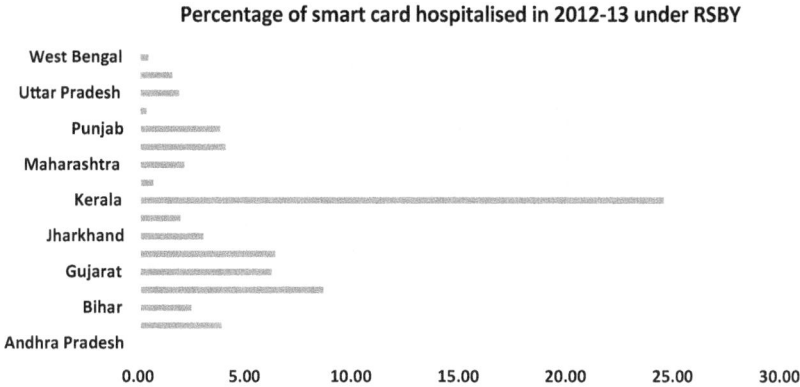

Figure 3.7 Hospitalisations by smart card holders of RSBY in 2012–13.
Source: Tables 3.17 and 3.18.

compared to outpatient expenses (4.5%) or medicines (4.85%). The poorer income sections in RSBY have indeed experienced a rise in catastrophic headcount, a conclusive proof that RSBY and other state run insurance programmes have failed to provide financial risk protection", the report noted. The report pointed out that a "major design flaw in RSBY and other such state health insurance programmes is their narrow focus on secondary and tertiary care hospitalisation. Essentially, these models are designed to address low-volume, high-value financial transactions that could result in catastrophic expenditure and impoverishment of households. However, evidence points in the opposite direction." The study also emphasised that RSBY utilisation was higher by people who already had better access to health care services, and the most marginalised sections were being excluded further.

A study by Patel and Patel (2016)[9] was conducted in 2013 in a coastal district of Odisha. It focussed on out-of-pocket expenditure (OOP) and utilisation of RSBY during hospital stays. According to the study, RSBY beneficiaries stated that public hospitals remain under-equipped in comparison to the private ones. But due to the scheme respondents were able to access costly medicines at both private and public hospital without spending out-of-pocket. In private hospitals however, beneficiaries had to spend extra money on travel to bring hard copies of supportive documents such as ID proof and also incurred high OOP payment when the INR 30,000 of RSBY coverage was exhausted. Complaints of rude behaviour of hospital staff were also attributed to the fact that they were RSBY beneficiaries. They felt RSBY creates a boundary between poor and rich people within private hospitals. The

Table 3.19 State-wise Total number of beneficiaries under RSBY (2008–2014)

Selected State-wise Number of Beneficiaries Availed Benefits under Rashtriya Swasthya Bima Yojana (RSBY) in India (2012–2013 and 2014–2015)

States/UTs	2008–09	2009–10	2010–11	2011–12	2012–13	2013–14	2014–15
Andhra Pradesh	-	-	-	-	255	255	-
Assam	69	-	7224	26,985	11,179	20,720	40,506
Bihar	-	37,060	98,570	294,383	244,715	171,450	5659
Chhattisgarh	-	2418	41,819	152,531	184,677	186,982	230,480
Goa	-	7	-	-	-	-	-
Gujarat	3286	68,392	50,402	125,958	157059	130,378	75,111
Haryana	3220	57,129	40,395	65,395	46,542	24,008	14,136
Jharkhand	305	15,599	35,061	52,001	50,580	64,887	57,005
Karnataka	-	-	1999	57,976	62,183	144	-
Kerala	149	133,618	380,422	518,871	637,942	674,681	295920
Madhya Pradesh	-	-	-	-	6045	8677	12,966
Maharashtra	4	31,648	30,887	88,808	61,040	13,854	-
Odisha	-	46	3792	127,465	247,555	112,525	313,197
Punjab	161	3896	8317	11,143	10,264	5948	9020
Rajasthan	664	-	-	-	3415	5305	11,080
Tamil Nadu	-	3721	1475	-	-	-	-
Uttar Pradesh	831	79,292	360,144	263,525	201,363	98,687	112,791
Uttarakhand	-	875	3522	20,473	10,371	6989	9763
West Bengal	140	9634	33,054	227,640	264,502	245,366	329,631
India	12,541	457,481	1,174,905	2,146,176	2362,450	1,947,231	1,676,334

Source: Lok Sabha Unstarred Question No. 5251, dated on 24.04.2015. Lok Sabha Unstarred Question No. 979, dated on 27.07.2015.

Table 3.20 State-wise Total number of Workers of unorganised sector benefitted under RSBY (2013–14)

Selected State-wise Number of Workers of Unorganised Sector Benefitted under Rashtriya Swasthya Bima Yojana (RSBY) in India (2013–2014 to 2015–2016)

States/UTs	2013–2014	2014–2015	2015–2016
Andhra Pradesh	2184	*	*
Assam	1,416,919	1,421,104	1,421,104
Bihar	6,102,774	818,531	6,888,208
Chhattisgarh	2,265,370	2,141,822	3,442,749
Gujarat	1,900,903	1,876,307	1,876,628
Haryana	465,797	437,850	437,850
Jharkhand	1,923,138	1,714,552	1,682,894
Karnataka	29,417	6,050,439	6,747,113
Kerala	3,662,511	2,018,764	2,021,572
Madhya Pradesh	608,748	608,748	*
Maharashtra	234,252	*	*
Odisha	4,238,040	4,307,538	4,462,959
Punjab	236,764	232,352	232,352
Rajasthan	2,511,663	2,692,626	2,769,097
Uttar Pradesh	5,541,225	3,839,765	1,464,242
Uttarakhand	285,435	285,435	285,229
West Bengal	5,748,689	6,063,390	6,150,716
India	38,515,411	35,927,971	41,258,416

Note: * Not Implemented. Source: Lok Sabha Unstarred Question No. 2109, dated on 06.05.2016.

study suggests that to realise the equity objectives of RSBY, empanelled hospitals must be well regulated.

Another study by Bandyopadhyay and Sen (2017)[10] reviews the economic viability of the Rashtriya Swasthya Bima Yojana (RSBY), in West Bengal. The study argues that the market failure conditions of this insurance model perpetuate losses for not only the state, but also for insurance companies, unless they adjust on a continuous basis for profit by raising the premium rate, and this will otherwise affect the long run viability of the scheme.

A study by Jain (2017)[11] points out several challenges for RSBY. The latter include limited benefits, absence of linkage with preventive and primary care, use of old BPL lists, absence of a national-level independent body to manage the scheme, difficulty in enrolling an additional member, lack of capacities at different levels, namely, building capacities needed at each level to run a health insurance programme, managing health care providers, building awareness, controlling fraud and doing data analytics.

Annexure 1

Table 3.A.1 Status of CGHS as on 2000

Status of Central Government Health Scheme (CGHS) in India (As on 31.03.2000)

Particulars	Number
Date of Commencement	1.7.1954 (Delhi)
No. of stations covered	18 (+2 at Ranchi and Bhubaneswar solely for AG's employees)
No. of card holders	986,877
No. of beneficiaries	4,237,088
No. of pensioners under CGHS	
Cards	182,110
Beneficiaries	577,805
Total no. of dispensaries	319
Allopathic dispensaries	241
Ayurvedic dispensaries/units	31
Homeopathic dispensaries/units	34
Unani dispensaries/units	9
Siddha dispensaries/units	2
Yoga centres	3
Polyclinics (including one at Kanpur being set up)	19
Laboratories	65
Dental units	17
Norms of expansion	6000 or more Central Government Employees and Pensioners
Norms of new dispensary	2000 or more Central Government Employees and Pensioners in a radius of 3 kms.

Source: MOHFW, GoI (1991).

Table 3.A.2 City-wise CGHS Dispensaries

Selected City-wise Number of Central Government
Health Scheme (CGHS) Dispensaries in India
(As on 13.02.2018)

City	Dispensaries		Poly	CGHS	Dental
	Allopathy	AYUSH	Clinic	Lab	Units
Agartala	1	-	-	-	-
Ahmedabad	8	2	1	1	1
Aizwal	1	-	-	-	-
Allahabad	7	2	1	1	0
Bangalore	10	4	1	3	1
Bhopal	2	0	0	0	0
Bhubaneswar	3	1		1	0
Chandigarh	1	-	-	-	0
Chennai	14	4	2	4	1
Dehradun	2	-	-	-	0
Delhi	95	36	4	34	6
Gandhinagar	1	-	-	-	-
Gangtok	1	-	-	-	-
Guwahati	5	1	-	-	0
Hyderabad	13	6	2	2	1
Imphal	1	-	-	-	-
Indore	1	-	-	-	-
Jabalpur	5	-	-	1	0
Jaipur	7	2	1	4	1
Jammu	2	-	-	-	0
Kanpur	9	3	-	3	1
Kohima	1	-	-	-	-
Kolkata	18	4	1	5	1
Lucknow	9	3	1	3	1
Meerut	6	2	0	2	1
Mumbai	26	5	2	4	3
Nagpur	11	3	1	1	1
Panaji	1	-	-	-	-
Patna	5	2	1	1	1
Puducherry	1	-	-	-	0
Pune	9	3	1	2	1
Raipur	1	-	0	0	0
Ranchi	3	-	-	1	-
Shillong	2	-	0	-	0
Shimla	1	-	-	-	0
Thiruvananthapuram	3	2	0	-	0
Visakhapatnam	1	-	-	-	0
India	**287**	**85**	**19**	**73**	**21**

Table 3.A.3 Empanelled Hospitals and Diagnostic Centre under CGHS

Selected City-wise Number of Hospitals and Diagnostic Centres Empanelled
under Central Government Health Scheme (CGHS) in India
(As on 30.11.2015)

Cities	Hospitals	Eye clinic	Dental clinic	Total	Diagnostic centre
Ahmedabad	10	4	1	15	1
Allahabad	25	4	8	37	5
Bangalore	14	33	4	51	5
Bhopal	13	2	Nil	15	3
Bhubaneshwar	10	1	1	12	Nil
Chandigarh	9	6	2	17	6
Chennai	16	6	2	24	5
Dehradun	8	4	Nil	12	4
Delhi	118	104	52	274	61
Guwahati	3	Nil	Nil	3	2
Hyderabad	69	16	6	91	5
Jabalpur	18	7	5	30	4
Jaipur	24	13	4	41	3
Jammu	Nil	1	Nil	1	Nil
Kanpur	39	9	1	49	10
Kolkata	8	4	Nil	12	15
Lucknow	20	13	3	36	10
Meerut	20	5	3	28	2
Mumbai	27	15	2	44	2
Nagpur	39	19	4	62	12
Patna	18	4	4	26	3
Pune	47	11	3	61	4
Ranchi	2	2	Nil	4	Nil
Shillong	Nil	Nil	Nil	Nil	Nil
Trivandrum	1	3	Nil	4	3
India	**558**	**286**	**105**	**949**	**165**

Source: Lok Sabha Starred Question No. 84, dated on 04.12.2015.

Table 3.A.4 Brief Description of Benefits, Contributory Conditions, Duration of Benefits and the Scale of Benefits of ESIS

Benefit	Contributory Condition	Duration	Rate
Sickness Benefit			
Sickness Benefit	Payment of contribution for 78 days in corresponding contribution period.	Up to 91 days in two consecutive benefit periods.	70% of the average daily wages.
Enhanced Sickness Benefit	Same as Above	14 days for Tubectomy& 7 days for vasectomy, extendable on medical advice	100% of the average daily wages
Extended Sickness Benefit	For 34 specified long-term diseases, continuous insurable employment for two years with minimum 156 days' contribution in four consecutive contribution periods.	124 days during a period of two years. This may be extended up to two years on medical advice.	80% of the average daily wages.
Disablement Benefit			
Temporary Disablement Benefit	From day one of entering insurable employment for disablement due to employment injury.	As long as temporary disablement lasts.	90% of the average daily wages approx.
Permanent Disablement Benefit	From day one of entering insurable employment for disablement due to employment injury.	For whole life	For permanent total disablement - 90% of average daily wages. For permanent partial disablement-proportionate to the loss of earning capacity as determined by the medical board.
Dependants' Benefit	From day one of entering insurable employment in case of death due to employment injury.	For life to the widow or until her re-marriage. To dependent children till the age of 25 years. To dependant parents etc. subject to conditions.	90% of average daily wages shareable in fixed proportion among all dependants.
Maternity Benefit	Payment of contribution of 70 days in two preceding contribution periods.	Up to 12 weeks in case of confinement. Up to 6 weeks in case of miscarriage. Extendable by 1 month on medical advice in case of sickness arising out of Pregnancy, Confinement, Miscarriage	100% of the average daily wages.

(Continued)

Table 3.A.4 (Continued)

Benefit	Contributory Condition	Duration	Rate
Medical Benefit	Reasonable medical facilities for self and family from day one of entering insurable employment.	Reasonable medical care till he/she remains in insurable employment	
Other Benefits			
Confinement Expenses	An Insured Woman or an IP in respect of his wife is eligible if confinement occurs at a place where necessary medical facilities under ESI Scheme are not available.	Up to two confinements only	Rs.5,000/-per case
Funeral Expenses	From day one of entering insurable employment	For defraying expenses on the funeral of an insured person	Actual expenses subject to a maximum of Rs.10,000/-
Vocational Training	In case of physical disablement due to employment injury	As long as vocational training lasts.	Actual fee charged or Rs.123/- a day, whichever is higher.
Physical Rehabilitation	In case of physical disablement due to employment injury	As long as person is admitted in an artificial limb centre.	100% of the average daily wages.
Unemployment Allowance (RGSKY)	In case of involuntarily loss of employment due to closure of factory, retrenchment or permanent invalidity due to non-employment injury and the contribution in respect of him have been paid/payable for a minimum of three years prior to the loss of employment	Maximum 12 months during lifetime	50% of the average daily wages
Skill Up gradation Training	Same as above.	For a duration of maximum 6 months.	

Source: *Employee State Insurance Corporation*, https://www.esic.nic.in/

Table 3.A.5 Income and Expenditure of Employees State Insurance Corporation (ESIC) in India (2001 to 2007, as on 31st March)

Particulars	2001	2002	2003	2004	2005	2006	2007
Income							
Contribution from Both Employers and Employees	125544	124991.4	130238.61	138,071.97	168,908.48	193,356.47	245,348.37
Interest and Dividends	24295.13	39727.95	32697.79	51334.11	48624.73	39839.26	57880.99
Rents, Rates, Taxes, Fees, Fines and Forfeitures	6034.98	6004.11	6204.45	6331.05	6113.42	6451.06	5791.96
Medical Education							
Miscellaneous	379.55	2154.65	781.2	1455.01	959.42	1414.98	1789.87
Expenditure							
Medical Benefit	54229.32	54337.44	56520.05	62038.29	68637.58	72411	77978.47
Cash Benefit	28563.78	30015.94	28561.37	27396.86	26469.02	27373.82	27231.39
Other Benefits	76.98	77.81	79.74	80.69	80.46	97.16	89.85
Administrative Expenses	17094.63	17643.52	17722	18277.01	19996.18	21096.22	22139.27
Provision for Depreciation of Hospitals etc., Repair and Maintenance and Reserve Funds	2016.23	2087.76	2436.62	9254.68	10636.29	6917.96	7425.41

(Continued)

Table 3.A.5 (Continued)

Particulars	2008	2009	2010	2012	2013
Income					
Contribution from Both Employers and Employees	326283.98	369853.27	389600.19	707011.20	811144.55
Interest and Dividends	62836.03	66327.23	111017.11	118802.36	191448.89
Rents, Rates, Taxes, Fees, Fines and Forfeitures	7898.75	7523.46	7154.72	8607.01	7650.15
Medical Education				67.51	151.51
Miscellaneous	1913.07	1541.74	745.91	2867.03	3467.00
Expenditure					
Medical Benefit	92479.29	112322.31	162693.06	268962.11	393190.74
Cash Benefit	28728.15	38070.45	42693.2	68185.03	76116.95
Other Benefits	209.4	252.3	189.5	320.79	261.47
Administrative Expenses	24797.39	41276.17	50436.47	64706.48	82610.84
Provision for Depreciation of Hospitals etc., Repair and Maintenance and Reserve Funds	8671.57	14961.75	15168.07	16925.23	12577.83

Source: Ministry of Labour and Employment, Govt. of India. (ON274) & (ON808)

Table 3.A.6 Selected State-wise Cash and Other Benefits under ESIS

Selected State-wise Cash and Other Benefits Given under Employees
State Insurance Act, 1948 in India - Part II
(2014–2015)

States/UTs	Sickness Benefits		Maternity Benefits		Dependants Benefits	
	No. of Fresh Claims	Total Amount Paid (Rs. in Lakh)	No. of Confine- ments	Total Amount Paid (Rs. in Lakh)	Total No. of Death Cases Admitted	Capitalised Value of Benefit Claims Admitted (Rs. in ' 000)
Andhra Pradesh						
Hyderabad	42407	1719	1881	59498724	97	99971721
Vijayawada	30283	714	578	14207245	22	23978982
Vishakhapatnam	18043	531	289	7269142	28	26822000
Assam Meghalaya Tripura	3854	106	216	4045126	20	13897321
Sikkim Nagaland						
Bihar	1650	56	55	860004	9	10076512
Chandigarh	1198	51	180	4574511	10	9224615
Chhattisgarh	6872	251	83	2007687	70	62886855
Delhi						
Rajendra Place	13124	409	298	9062901	22	34809989
Okhla	2958	215	196	5503650	25	30190924
Rohini	3121	228	90	2490321	27	30948357
Goa	7572	217	390	11367239	15	12643440
Gujarat						
Ahmedabad	17044	582	327	7668197	85	76529263
Vadodara	6799	319	84	2724619	40	35797677
Surat	3058	153	167	4036523	47	44139454
Haryana						
Faridabad	5853	392	933	27241065	116	110744804
Gurgaon	1479	224	312	7617810	45	54713438
Ambala	1455	57	58	1469937	16	14031748
Himachal Pradesh	9010	328	269	5469024	15	9684923
Jammu and Kashmir	1811	83	84	1763273	20	21728485
Jharkhand	11356	315	144	3156403	25	24517919
Karnataka						
Bangalore Mysore Mangalore	16847	617	1922	37598680	31	27271092
Bomasundra	8758	360	1691	38165460	10	5952586
Peenya	16133	609	1770	32953256	13	14836508
Hubli	16765	546	315	6772520	19	19126909
Gulbarga	4311	138	61	1045023	5	2643564
Mysore	10594	270	275	6749293	21	101824456
Mangalore	6018	171	693	17043635	5	4185853

(Continued)

Table 3.A.6 (Continued)

Selected State-wise Cash and Other Benefits Given under Employees State Insurance Act, 1948 in India - Part II (2014–2015)

Kerala					
Kerala Trichur	33374	527	868	326084655	7	7968621
Ernakulam	41423	1060	2656	72397220	22	34495513
Kollam, Thiruvananthapuram	26494	761	1519	33708670	14	14334213
Kozhikode	6367	422	672	28680245	9	11084513
Thiruvananthapuram	5823	262	1275	33575458	3	1502336
Madhya Pradesh	34533	860	422	8636571	56	42875490
Maharashtra						
Lower Parel	5879	358	662	20438418	29	36023001
Marol	9960	395	1346	34171102	19	20249583
Nagpur	13721	431	108	3335913	23	22012635
Pune, Nasik	36935	880	583	15969599	33	49594815
Thane	9007	321	645	16407280	23	22808815
Aurangabad	7583	234	54	1349292	7	8021947
Nasik	2114	215	57	4933789	27	37801768
Odisha	9904	419	286	5342009	49	32946336
Puducherry						
YenamMahe	11098	232	451	9979695	13	6475710
Punjab	6930	262	375	8578645	44	34831679
Ludhiana	4182	316	240	5710614	27	23514600
Jallandhar	6895	240	206	4752888	24	19504364
Rajasthan						
Jaipur	9001	324	267	6089504	86	74178341
Udaipur, Jodhpur	4119	161	160	3352427	25	20735639
Jodhpur	3893	192	62	1505577	25	23727591
Tamil Nadu						
Chennai	10112	936	1996	75891679	110	109943319
Coimbatore	6706	297	1153	32814740	55	54157131
Madurai	4923	253	1052	18677382	58	42326355
Salem	3537	142	587	12600053	28	21068771
Tirunelveli	3242	146	502	10446828	9	6607555
Uttar Pradesh						
Kanpur	7815	264	79	1943708	67	54636935
Noida	2507	75	424	9519184	111	136261723
Varanasi	6988	384	13	283668	6	4557075
Lucknow	237	10	50	1007382	13	9637682
Uttarakhand	6792	303	197	6087192	21	14317164
West Bengal						
Kolkata	49475	2693	465	11960496	52	49231474
Barrackpore	13965	922	54	1006900	25	29112350
Durgapur	4373	167	27	615930	33	31610744
Meghalaya	0	0	0	0	0	0
India	**668282**	**25125**	**32874**	**850215981**	**2020**	**1940335183**

Source: Ministry of Labour and Employment, Govt. of India. (ON1374)

Table 3.A.7 Selected State-wise Other Benefits Given under ESIS

Selected State-wise Cash and Other Benefits Given under Employees
State Insurance Act, 1948 in India - Part I
(2014–2015)

States/UTs	Attendance at Dispensaries in Respect of Insured Persons	No. of Cases Admitted in Hospitals	Disablement Benefits		
			Claims Admitted	Amount of Temporary Disablement Benefit Paid (Rs. in '000)	Capitalised Value of Permanent Disablement Benefit Claims Admitted (Rs. in '000)
Andhra Pradesh					
Hyderabad	1120593	154933	1461	19492	70235600
Vijayawada	0	-	770	6308	25322100
Vishakhapatnam	0	-	1310	13276	17731100
Assam Meghalaya Tripura Sikkim Nagaland	178724	7356	163	2049	5599300
Bihar	55164	4383	257	8257	8252500
Chandigarh	85630	63956	75	1422	4634000
Chhattisgarh	313531	0	422	6692	31608600
Delhi					
Rajendra Place	1790092	122230	375	13643	62664200
Okhla	0	9270	75	2491	10538000
Rohini	0	-	701	23384	82997800
Goa	123300	-	202	2953	5995100
Gujarat					
Ahmedabad	1132264	69005	4800	34487	72720800
Vadodara	0	-	909	9715	14721900
Surat	0	-	290	4811	34239800
Haryana					
Faridabad + Ambala	0	0	1590	21469	135165700
Gurgaon	0	-	284	7792	73097760
Ambala	0	-	438	5314	47156400
Himachal Pradesh	74231	109314	729	8955	35028700
Jammu and Kashmir	0	0	336	3039	10463000
Jharkhand	15567	19631	279	4810	22597400
Karnataka					
Bangalore Mysore Mangalore	3103750	451422	618	7914	25540000
Bomasundra	0	-	192	2370	4852500
Peenya	0	663	6377	21455300	
Hubli	0	-	1673	11235	22456000
Gulbarga	0	-	94	1041	2566400
Mysore	0	0	398	3815	34143200
Mangalore	0	0	134	1831	1052500
Kerala Trichur	2697974	263250	1372	7299	7795000
Ernakulam	0	-	1840	20378	28245000
Kollam, Thiruvananthapuram	0	-	1208	10895	21136606

(Continued)

Table 3.A.7 (Continued)

Selected State-wise Cash and Other Benefits Given under Employees
State Insurance Act, 1948 in India - Part I
(2014–2015)

Kozhikode	0	-	110	109511	11638900
Thiruvananthapuram	0	-	197	2762	9807500
Madhya Pradesh	829407	56059	4172	22770	89594700
Maharashtra					
Lower Parel	528964	80030	133	2495	13628000
Marol	0	-	376	4877	22429200
Nagpur	-	-	936	9053	7944400
Pune, Nasik	-	-	2084	23252	100528900
Thane	-	-	768	8627	47140100
Aurangabad	-	-	469	4115	3079700
Nasik	-	-	415	8333	82667200
Odisha	0	0	576	7765	8109800
Puducherry					
YamanMahe	114395	49440	258	3565	11067400
Punjab	1085114	53311	1069	15538	65983100
Ludhiana	0	-	1885	27606	138411700
Jallandhar	0	-	549	7130	31072800
Rajasthan					
Jaipur	1119988	71918	1003	11131	66914000
Udiapur, Jodhpur	-	-	864	6780	14980700
Jodhpur	-	-	437	5893	28460900
Tamil Nadu					
Chennai	4394928	188136	1092	19035	71184300
Coimbatore	0	41712	740	8935	38269406
Madurai	-	-	420	4223	24094900
Salem	-	-	327	3431	14800000
Tirunelveli	-	-	195	2054	9689600
Uttar Pradesh					
Kanpur	308930	0	338	5838	23765100
Noida	-	-	663	10298	79287800
Varanasi	-	-	14	387	0
Lucknow	-	-	149	2104	2287600
Uttarakhand	248970	0	542	7714	6519200
West Bengal					
Kolkata	2127498	33262	25880	322675	139663200
Barrackpore	-	-	7796	134565	124171700
Durgapur	0	-	332	4255	17856500
Meghalaya	8994	0	0	0	0
India	**21598098**	**1848618**	**78647**	**981673**	**2245060500**

Source: Ministry of Labour and Employment, Govt. of India. (ON1374)

Table 3.A.8 Families Enrolled under RSBY (2012–17, States and All India)

Selected State-wise Number of BPL Families Covered under Rashtriya Swasthya Bima Yojana (RSBY) in India; 2012–2013 to 2016–2017

States/UTs	2012–2013		2013–2014		2014–2015		2015–2016		2016–2017	
	BPL Target	BPL Enrolled	BPL Target	BPL Enrolled	BPL Target	BPL Enrolled	BPL Target	BPL Enrolled	BPL Target	BPL Enrolled
Andhra Pradesh	-	2184	-	2184	-	*	-	*	-	-
Arunachal Pradesh	23888	14158								
Assam	361036	176906	2522563	1416919	2676874	1421104	2704907	1421104	2371950	1421104
Bihar	13102868	7634503	11177403	6102774	6790986	818531	11106552	6899144 *	13921372	7028409
Chandigarh	-	-	9548	5854	20223	7865			-	-
Chhattisgarh	3317598	2285345	3325418	1962689	3882032	2141822	3203437	3442749	4869167	4146227
Delhi	987824	95597								
Gujarat	3799976	1883179	4509836	1900903	4816150	1876307	4570183	1876628	4653237	2691497
Haryana	1280714	560241	1317101	463226	1229850	437850	1257051	437850		
Himachal Pradesh	479919	286492	572886	341818	736575	481699 *	704736	480588 *	877763	480588
Jammu and Kashmir	66005	35521	17537	4988						
Jharkhand	2812898	1462235	4303118	1923138	3968109	1714552	3832366	1682894		
Karnataka	4027038	1650271	320029	29417	11088340	6050439	11088340	6731881	10031663	6206620
Kerala	3283478	2743665	3840895	2747029	2217954	2018764	2221283	2021572 *	2275705	2060953
Madhya Pradesh	293937	116510	1102589	608748	1191258	608748 *		*		
Maharashtra	3436269	1747157	4911911	234252						
Manipur	110173	66753	120225	68140	120237	70383	106058	70925	120237	70925
Meghalaya	168705	78395	218469	108321	218469	65840	218469	256138	479743	256138
Mizoram	221814	103545	333211	145842	212572	152983	156677	152983 *	243407	194886
Nagaland	322927	143585	407365	151806	468055	128184			518476	255314
Odisha	5221931	3388096	5683766	4238040	6538381	4307538	6548999	4462959 *	6158498	4462959
Puducherry	15142	9486	15142	9486	18724	6467				
Punjab	477613	226878	454070	236764	454255	232352	454255	232352		
Rajasthan	1075380	732889	3418503	2511663	3768380	2692626	3829760	2769097		
Tripura	786913	505327	786913	505327	775930	505327	333994	492022	768359	481331
Uttar Pradesh	11091220	5396503	11093457	5541225	9343930	3839765	5390145	285229		
Uttarakhand	736953	334694	746197	285435	821119	285435	822428	1464242	728216	285229
West Bengal	9036747	5766731	9371984	5748689	11127061	6063390	11127061	6150716	11100347	6290446
India	66538966	37446846	66159416	37294677	72485464	35927971	69676701	41331073	59118140	36332626

Note: States not implementing RSBY during the period. Source: Lok Sabha Unstarred Question No. 21, dated on 07.07.2014; Lok Sabha Unstarred Question No. 106, dated on 03.03.2015, Lok Sabha Unstarred Question No. 979, dated on 27.07.2015,Lok Sabha Unstarred Question No. 1746, dated on 10.03.2017 &Lok Sabha Unstarred Question No. 2192, dated on 28.07.2017.

Annexure 2

New Initiatives under Health Reform Agenda of ESIC also have added other functions by ESIS

Electronic Health Records of ESI beneficiaries: The Health Records of the ESI Beneficiaries (Insured Persons and their family members) has been made available online now. The records also include laboratory reports in digital form and there will be no need to visit the hospital for getting the required information.

Abhiyan Indradhanush: This is a manifestation of the Swachh Bharat Abhiyan in ESIC and has been implemented in all the ESIS Hospitals ensuring the change of bedsheets daily as per VIBGYOR pattern.

A 24x7 Toll Fee Medical Helpline No. 1800-11-3839 has been set up for attending the calls of Insured persons and their Family members who wish to seek advice and guidance from casualty/emergency of ESIC Hospitals.

Special OPD for Sr. Citizens and Differently-abled Persons in ESIC Hospitals has been started for hassle-free treatment.

AYUSH: The AYUSH facilities has been extended to all ESIC Dispensaries and Hospitals.

Other salient features of Health Reforms Agenda:

Extending Coverage: ESI scheme is being implemented in the remaining north-east states of Arunachal Pradesh, Mizoram, Manipur and Andaman & Nicobar Islands by 31.12.2015

Health Scheme is being opened for selected group and unorganised workers like Rickshaw Pullers/Auto Rickshaw drivers in selected urban/metropolitan areas on pilot basis.

ESI coverage has been extended to construction site workers in the implemented areas w.e.f 01.08.2015.

ESI Scheme is being implemented in Industrial/Commercial clusters of the whole of 393 districts of the states.

Improving Patients / Attendant Care:

Appropriate Cancer detection/treatment, cardiology and dialysis facilities in all the ESIC Hospitals have been provided on PPP Mode.

A special Focus has been made for upgradation of 24 dispensaries to 30 bedded set up for providing 24x7 services in first phase.

New Initiatives ESIS.

Pathological and X-ray facilities will be provided in all the Dispensaries on PPP Mode in Phases. Pathological, Laboratory and ECG Services have been started in ESI Dispensary of Delhi/Noida area from November 2015.

The tele-medicine project is expected to go live shortly in all the ESIC Hospitals.

For better management for helping in registration and Pharmacy, an effective queue management system is implemented in all hospitals. To establish better rapport between doctors and patients, doctors, para medical and other staff are given behavioural training periodically. The system of collecting feedback form all indoor patients is already available in all hospitals. Reception and "May I Help You" facilities in each hospital to guide the patients/attendants are also available.

Cleanliness drive in all ESIC Hospital under Swachh Bharat Abhiyan:

ESIC is taking special care to keep its hospitals neat and clean. As a part of National Drive of Swachh Bharat Abhiyan, The ESI Corporation has launched 2nd Phase of special Cleanliness Drive since June 22 2015. All the ESIC Hospitals have been directed to complete white-washing and painting of the building along with minor repair before Deepawali festival this year. The hospitals have been directed to improve the horticulture on their premises. Flowerpots are to be installed in the internal areas also for improving the ambience. All service areas in the hospitals will be well lit. Paper rolls may be used on the examination bed in the doctor's chambers. Cleanliness of toilets have been given importance. The concerned Medical Superintendents have been asked to make arrangements for morning and evening monitoring.

Tracking of every pregnant mother & newborn: With a view to ensure 100 per cent immunisation as well as safe delivery, every mother and newborn child of Insured Persons, a pilot project for tracking every pregnant mother and new born is to be started in Delhi, for which coordination is being done with the state Programme Officer under Ministry of Health and Family Welfare.

Mother and Childcare Hospitals in every state: ESIC has constituted a committee to prepare the norms for setting up a Mother and Childcare Hospital in every state.

AYUSH

Besides Allopathic treatment, ESIC Hospitals also provide treatment under AYUSH (Ayurveda, Yoga, Unani, Siddha and Homeopathy). Ayurveda facility is available in 30 ESIC Hospitals and 9 ESIC Dispensaries and Homeopathy in 12 ESIC Hospitals and 5 ESIC Dispensaries and Yoga in 6 ESIC Hospitals. Facility of AYUSH is to be extended to all dispensaries in phases by December 2015 and Yoga in all ESIC Hospitals by November 30, 2015

Notes

1 A list of these MDGs are presented in Annexure 1 to this chapter
2 Also Capital expenditure are mentioned separately only for Social Health Insurance Schemes. Cash benefits for sickness, maternity, disablement, and death due to injury at work to workers and dependents to cover for wage loss or other means are not included within the boundary of NHA for India. Interest paid on revenues, dividends, reserves of the insurer (after claims are paid including administrative over heads) are also outside the health insurance expenditures boundary and are not generally mentioned under health insurance expenditure.
3 http://pib.nic.in/newsite/PrintRelease.aspx?relid=106436
4 A detailed list of benefits under ESIS is presented in Annexure1 Table 4 to this Chapter
5 A government officer (called Field Key Officer – FKO) needs to be present and must insert his/ her own, government-issued smart card to verify the legitimacy of the enrolment. (In this way, each enrolee can be tracked to a particular state government official). In addition to the FKO, an insurance company representative/ smart card agency representative must be present. At the end of each day of enrolment, the list of households which have been issued smart cards is sent to the state nodal agency. This list of enrolled households is maintained centrally and is the basis for financial transfers from the Government of India to the state governments.
6 If a diagnosis leads to a hospitalization, the assistant at the help desk checks whether the procedure is in the list of pre-specified packages. If the procedure is in the list, the appropriate prescribed package is selected from the menu. If the procedure is not in the package list, the help desk assistant checks with the insurer regarding the price for that procedure. Upon release of the beneficiary from the hospital, the card is again swiped along with fingerprint verification and the pre-specified cost of the procedure is deducted from the amount available on the card. The beneficiary is also paid by the hospital Rs. 100 as transportation expense at the time of the discharge. However, total transportation assistance cannot exceed Rs. 1000/- per year and it is part of Rs. 30,000/- coverage. No proof is required to be submitted by the beneficiary to get the transportation
7 Information relating to transactions that take place each day at each hospital is sent through a phone line to a district server. A separate set of pre-formatted tables are generated for the insurer and for the government respectively. This allows the insurer to track claims, transfer funds to the hospitals and investigate in the case of suspicious claim patterns through on-site audits.
8 Council for Social Development, "India: Social Development Report 2014." New Delhi
9 Patel Gupteswar and Patel Kripalini (2016), Op-25: Rastriya Swasthya Bima Yojana and Health Equity: User Experiences and Reflections from Odisha (7 July, 2016); June 2016 - Volume 1 - Suppl 1.
10 Bandyopadhyay Satarupa and Kasturi Sen (2017), Challenges of Rasthryia Swasthya Bima Yojana (RSBY) in West Bengal, India: An exploratory study, The International Journal of Health Planning and Management Volume 33, Issue 2, First published: 20 October 2017;Pages: 294-308; https://doi.org/10.1002/hpm.2453
11 Jain, Nishant. August 2017. *Role of Government-funded and Community-based Health Insurance Schemes in Moving toward Universal Health Coverage in India.* Bethesda, MD: Health Finance & Governance Project, Abt Associates Inc.

References

Ahmad, Nabi (2001). "A study of the working of Employees State Insurance Corporation and its impact on Social Security in India." Thesis Submitted under Department of Commerce Aligarh Muslim University Aligarh (India).

Chattopadhyay, A., T. Mondal, T. K. Saha, I. Dey, B. K. Sahu, and J. Bhattacharya (2013). "An audit of prescribing practices in CGHS dispensaries of Kolkata, India." *IOSR-JDMS* 8: 32–37.

Chowdhury, J. A. (2006). "Comparison of the health sector in India, Indonesia and Thailand: Policy prescription for India." Independent Commission on Development and Health in India. New Delhi: Voluntary Health Association of India. Available at http://www.vhai.org/ceo/icdhi-publications/Comparison%20of%20the%20Health%20Sector%20in%20India,%20Indonesia%20and%20Thailand.pdf.

Dash, U. and V. R. Muraleedharan (2011). "How equitable is employees' state insurance scheme in India?: A case study of Tamil Nadu." The Consortium for Research on Equitable Health Systems (CREHS) and Indian Institute of Technology (Madras), India June.

Devadasan, N., ed. (2006). Planning and implementing health insurance programmes in India: An operational guide. Bangalore: Institute of Public Health India. Available at http://www.ilo.org/gimi/gess/ShowRessource.action?ressource.ressourceId=337 (accessed on 30 November 2014).

Employee State Insurance Corporation https://www.esic.nic.in/.

GoI (2013). Report No.71, *The Functioning of Central Government Health Scheme (CGHS)*, (Ministry of Health and Family Welfare), Parliament of India, Department-Related Parliamentary Standing Committee, Rajya Sabha August, (Presented to the Rajya Sabha on 6th August 2013), (Laid on the Table of Lok Sabha on 6th August, 2013), Rajya Sabha Secretariat, New Delhi.

GOI (2008). Standing Committee on Labour and Employment The Employees' State Insurance (Amendment) Bill, 2008, Thirty Sixth Report.

GOI, Planning Commission. Mid-term appraisal of the tenth five year plan (2002–2007). Available at http://planningcommission.gov.in/plans/mta/midterm/cont_eng1.htm (accessed on 30 November 2014).

Gumber, A. (2002). "Health insurance for the informal sector: Problems and prospects." New Delhi: Indian Council for Research on International Economic Relations. Available at http://icrier.org/pdf/WP-90.pdf (accessed on 30 November 2014).

Haldar, D., A. Sarkar, S. Bisoi, and P. Mondal (2008). "Assessment of client's perception in terms of satisfaction and service utilization in the central government health scheme dispensary at Kolkata." *Indian Journal of Community Medicine* 33: 121–123.

Jose, Mathew (2006). "A study on the working of the Employees' State Insurance Corporation." Thesis submitted to the Faculty of Commerce, Mahatma Gandhi University in partial fulfilment of the requirements for the award of the Degree of Doctor of Philosophy in Commerce.

Kumari, Aparajita, Nalin Ranjan Tripathy, and Amand Bhaskar (2016). "Central Government Health Services (CGHS) in perspective of beneficiaries satisfaction." *International Journal of Health Sciences & Research* 6(1): 401–409.

NPH (2018). "National Health Profile". Ministry of Health and Family Welfare.

Sarwal, Rakesh (2015). "Reforming central government health scheme into a 'Universal Health Coverage' model." *The National Medical Journal of India* 28(1): e1–e9.

Vellakkal, S., S. Juyal, and A. Mehdi (2010). "Healthcare delivery and stakeholder's satisfaction under social health insurance schemes in India: An evaluation of Central Government Health Scheme (CGHS) and Ex-servicemen Contributory Health Scheme (ECHS)." New Delhi: Indian Council for Research on International Economic Relations. Available at http://saber.eaber.org/node/23183 (accessed on 30 November 2014).

Chapter 4

Ayushman Bharat (MODI Care) and Other Government-Sponsored Health Insurance in India

Introduction

In this chapter, we focus on one of the recent budgetary interventions in the healthcare sector in India. Primarily, keeping the discussion on the much cherished goal of MODI Care, overall, a comparative profile of existing RSBY (Rashtriya Swasthya Bima Yojana), other state-sponsored health insurance schemes as well as potential pros and cons of MODI Care are highlighted from the national health perspective. Our analysis suggests that the new initiative by the central government in India could go a long way in reducing inequality in healthcare in India.

The per capita public expenditure on health in India is relatively very low. This is evident if we compare the Indian scenario with other countries in South Asia. Including central and state levels, public expenditure on health in India varied between Rs. 210 (in Bihar, a low-income state) to Rs. 1838 (in Goa, a high income state). Also, in terms of 2009–2010 constant prices, the inequity coefficients across 16 major Indian states indicated a Gini coefficient of .2780 and Thiel's entropy measure as .1280 for public expenditure on health. Even in terms of the state's own budgetary expenditure (in the range of Rs. 115 to 1696 at current prices), the Gini and entropy coefficient depicted values as .3129 and .2245.

Notably, central government expenditure through grants and off budget activities seemed to be more equitable. These amounts were in the range of Rs. 96 to 142 (from Bihar to Goa) and Gini and Thiel values were .225 and .082 respectively. However, the inequity in health infrastructure seemed to be high and the relevant inequity coefficient has gone up pertaining to three tiers of primary, secondary and tertiary care (Purohit, 2017).

Comparative Framework of Government Sponsored Health Insurance Schemes in India

Thus, keeping in mind the impact of Central government expenditure in the healthcare sector in India, this chapter builds around the possible equity impact of Central government schemes, specifically the health insurance

DOI: 10.4324/9781032615660-4

related schemes initiated by the Central budget. We will carry out a review of the existing literature that pertains to existing central government or state government health insurance schemes. This is followed by indicating major features of existing central and state insurance initiatives, which are at present operating in many of the Indian states. We will point out the gaps in these schemes and various merits, demerits and limitations of these initiatives. Finally, we will focus on the latest Central government initiative known as Ayushman Bharat, nicknamed as MODI CARE.

Literature Review

Concerning the healthcare insurance particularly relating to India, a number of research studies have analysed schemes, both centrally sponsored, or state government funded. We will attempt to look into the major studies that indicate the merits and demerits of existing governmental insurance schemes in India. The objective is to find lacunae or merits of these schemes from this review.

For instance, a study by Chauhan (2017) observed that the awareness level of unorganized workers (unskilled and semi-skilled) regarding the health insurance schemes is very poor. The study suggested that the health department should do the policymaking and ensure that every unorganized worker should be a member of a health insurance scheme within a period. It should also conduct awareness programme campaigns at specific times and places at regular intervals and insurance companies. NGOs can adopt localities to conduct awareness campaigns. It pointed out that at present nearly 86 per cent are unaware about health insurance schemes.

Sood et al. (2014) carried out a study on the implementation of a health insurance program (Vajpayee Arogyashree scheme) in the northern districts of Karnataka in India. It indicated that due to the scheme there was a reduction of 64 per cent in mortality among people below the poverty line, substantial reductions in out-of-pocket costs among beneficiaries and an increase in utilization. It opined that automatic enrolment of all below poverty line cardholders with no premiums removed the barriers to avail insurance and care, and the pre-authorization process mitigated the risk of overprovision of care. In addition, the services covered by the scheme were well matched to reflect conditions with a rising share of disease burden in India. Venkitasubramanian (2010) looked into PPP's model of health insurance in India. It observed that combining the Yeshaswini and Aarogyasri would be best for a social health insurance scheme. It suggested the creation of a Central Agency to strengthen the healthcare system and increase outsourcing to private players. It also suggested involvement of local authorities and co-operatives in premium collection and emphasized self-sustainability of the scheme. The suggested system could be a public-private partnership. Tejal and Ghosh (2018) pointed out that lack of targeting the truly needy and regulation of the private sector are also neglected in the Ayushman Bharat. Thus, the scheme will only help growth of the private sector in the secondary and tertiary care segments. Ahlin, Nichter and Pillai (2016) noted that most of the state insurance projects focus on in-patient hospital costs, not the larger burden of outpatient costs. They argued that ethnographic case studies could add much to existing health service and policy research and provide a better understanding of the life cycle and impact of insurance programs on both insurance holders and healthcare providers. Using fieldwork data from South India they identified areas such as public awareness, misunderstanding of insurance and health care utilization, behavior patterns in cash and cashless insurance systems, impact of insurance on quality of care and doctor-patient relations, health insurance coverage of chronic illnesses, rehabilitation and out of pocket (OOP) expenses which could be dealt in detail by researchers.

Nagaraju (2014) found a correlation between awareness and type of scheme, family coverage and receipt of smart card. The correlation coefficients of awareness for the total sum assured, coverage to family, inclusion procedures, eligibility conditions and preauthorization formalities is positive and significant. On the other hand, there is no significant correlation between the type of Scheme and awareness about the period, sum assured at credit, empanelled hospitals and types of diagnosis, diseases and follow up procedures covered. The number of family members covered under the Insurance Scheme has no significant relationship with the awareness of any aspects. However, the receipt of biometric cards and awareness of all the aspects of the Insurance Scheme correlate positively. It emphasized that the Government Sponsored Health Insurance Schemes should also follow tenets of potential Universal Health Care concepts. Thomas and Sakthi Vel (2011) evaluated emerging business models in private health insurance in India. It observed drawbacks such as a lack of standard terminology, protocol in treatment and billing of common illnesses. Different hospitals across the country even use differing terms, treatment protocols and charges for treating the same medical condition. Rathi (2017) observed that a huge informal sector in India remains uncovered by any health insurance scheme. Uneven income levels create difficulties to categorize and charge different premiums, as does the large rural population that is inaccessible and uninformed. Incongruent government policies impact upon various schemes and thus a comprehensive health insurance scheme could provide universal health coverage to the whole population.

Shekhar (2016) indicated that the design of the current social protection programs in the country lays heavy emphasis on hospital and specialty care and neglects to include primary healthcare. The study emphasized primary healthcare, inclusion of ambulatory care and its gate keeping function, coupled with primary healthcare screenings, to reduce the burden on the exchequer owing to costly tertiary and specialty services. This study also provides a synoptic feature view of central and state-sponsored schemes that exist in India.[1]

The study by Forgia and Nagpal (2012) observed that over 300 million people, or more than 25 per cent of India's population, gained access to some form of health insurance by 2010. It provides a comprehensive understanding of health insurance in India. The study points out that the new generation of Government Sponsored Health Insurance Schemes (GSHISs) is introducing explicit entitlements, improving accountability, and leveraging private capacity, particularly with an aim of reaching the poor. The recent health insurance initiatives by the government (central or state) create a mechanism of involving private sector hospitals in India. However, in these schemes, coverage is not comprehensive and is mostly focused on inpatient, often surgical, care. There are several operational constraints such as quality, cost containment, consumer protection and monitoring and evaluation. The report thus provides recommendations to address these issues, drawing on both Indian and international experience. It also recommends how GSHISs can improve the performance of primary care centres and their linkages with secondary and tertiary facilities. The study by Rajasekhar and Manjula (2012) carried out a comparative study of the health insurance schemes in Karnataka. It covered three major health insurance schemes in Karnataka and compared these to explore possibilities for convergence and synergy. The study used both primary and secondary data sources. Primary data was collected from field visits in three districts, namely, Shimoga, Bangalore Rural and Gulbarga. The districts of Shimoga and Bangalore (Rural) helped to study Yeshasvini and RSBY, while Gulbarga data was used for comparing Arogyasri and Yeshasvini schemes in the same setting. The study found duplication in the efforts made by the health insurance scheme for the poor in Karnataka, and indicated that the prime objective of 'equity, integrity and quality in health care' enshrined in the health policy of Karnataka government is not met. Thus, it suggested an integrated scheme to overcome the problems and procedures in the existing state-sponsored schemes.

Sarwal (2015) relied on publicly available documents to identify key features of universal health coverage (UHC) and relate it to the architecture of and practices in CGHS. It constructed a 'UHC status tool' of key elements and expected norms of UHC. The study concluded that it is both possible and desirable to transform CGHS into a UHC model within the same fiscal space. Garg (2014) highlighted the challenges in the management of health of informal workers. It suggested that health security for informal workers needs to be improved. It could be with some measures. These may include, for instance: mandatory insurance ensured by the employers for their employees, expansion of geographical and population coverage for the existing state schemes to cover informal workers that fall mainly in marginal and vulnerable categories, removal of supply side barriers to treatment, rehabilitation services for the poor, education and awareness to reduce demand-side barriers, safe work practices and improved surveillance and notification of occupational diseases. The study by Choudhury and Srinivasan (2011) indicates that four broad categories of insurance schemes are supported by Government of India that include crop insurance, life and group accident insurance, health insurance schemes against unforeseen health expenditure and livestock and sheep insurance schemes. At the state-level, the extent of overlap between Central and State schemes in terms of target groups and benefits appears to be small. In States like Andhra Pradesh, state-level schemes have also been merged with Central schemes to avoid overlap and extend a wider coverage to the poorer sections. Similarly, in Rajasthan and Karnataka, there are schemes where the Central and State schemes do not operate in the same districts to avoid overlapping. In the case of health insurance, although both the Universal Health Insurance Scheme (UHIS) and the Rashtriya Swasthya Bima Yojana provide insurance cover to the BPL population against hospitalization expenses, the UHIS is likely to be less relevant in the presence of RSBY as there is no requirement of premium contribution in RSBY. Presuming that, a substantial share of the Government's future expenditure commitment is likely to be directed towards the Rashtriya Swasthya Bima Yojana. The study points out some issues such as higher premium rates in RSBY relative to schemes like Aarogyashri in Andhra Pradesh, the weak institutional mechanism for monitoring the scheme and the limited scope of capital market solutions to providing insurance thus restricting the catastrophe bonds (CAT) use which have been used in other countries.

The study by Jain (2013) looked at four different health schemes operating in India. Each of these schemes are financed differently. Across all of the above differences, this paper has shown that health schemes that are rooted in highly unequal societies are likely to reproduce that inequality. However, it suggests integration of the health insurance schemes with the programmes that seek to improve living and working conditions more generally to reduce further inequity. The RSBY has not been based on a solid ground of equity and scant attention is paid to the state provision of basic primary healthcare. Further, the major focus of health insurance schemes in India is hospital-based care. Most of the schemes do not provide coverage for outpatient care or the cost of drugs. This leaves a big gap in their objective of preventing impoverishment due to health care. Yet in a little over three years, the RSBY has provided hospital-based insurance coverage to about 100 million people in a challenging and complex political and administrative environment, and it is laudable. The study also emphasized an increase in awareness pertaining to RSBY and other health insurances. Sharma et al. (2018) review the status of oral health care in India and indicate it to be a major public health concern. The review concludes that existing schemes appear to be pro-poor and are inclusive of disadvantaged minorities, the scheme suffers from adverse selection. These schemes have the potential to play an important role in India's move toward universal health coverage.

The study by Nandi, Schneider and Dixit (2017) focuses on RSBY in Chhattisgarh State in 2012. This study examined enrolment, utilization (public and private) and out of pocket (OOP) expenditure for the insured and uninsured, in Chhattisgarh. Both descriptive and multivariate analyses of factors associated with enrolment, hospitalization (by sector) and OOP expenditure were conducted, taking into account gender, socio-economic status, residence, type of facility and ailment. They found that 95.1 per cent of insured private sector users and 66.0 per cent of insured public sector users still incurred costs. Median OOP payments in the private sector were eight times those in the public sector. Of households with at least one member hospitalized, 35.5 per cent experienced catastrophic health expenditures (>10 per cent monthly household consumption expenditure). The study found that despite insurance coverage, the majority still incurred OOP expenditure. It suggests the need to further examine the roles of public and private sectors in financial risk protection through government health insurance.

The study by Sakthivel and Karan (2012) provides evidence on the impact of publicly financed health insurance schemes on financial risk protection in India's health sector. It conclusively demonstrates that the poorer sections of households in intervention districts of the Rashtriya Swasthya Bima Yojna, Rajiv Aarogyasri of Andhra Pradesh and Tamil Nadu Health Insurance schemes experienced a rise in real per capita healthcare expenditure, particularly on hospitalization, and an increase in catastrophic headcount. Thus, there is a conclusive proof that RSBY and other state government-based interventions failed to provide financial risk protection. The study applies a pre-insurance and post-insurance approach that involves the period 2004–2005 and 2009–2010, respectively, and it used a case-control approach.

Thus, above studies suggest that existing public sector health insurance mechanisms including RSBY and state-sponsored schemes have either one or more of the problems such as the overlapping of central and state insurance schemes, duplication of efforts by the same or different tier of governments, neglect of primary care and its role as gatekeeper, inpatient focus and neglect of out of pocket expenditure, lack of awareness among people, increasing roles to private empanelled hospitals, inequity and adverse section and lack of clarity about occupational and oral health care.

Main Features, Merits and Demerits and Gaps in Major Central and State Health care Insurance Schemes in India

In the light of the above review of literature, it is observed that the existing major centrally sponsored scheme, namely RSBY, is marked by its lower coverage, with an insurance cover of Rs.30,000 for a family comprising of at most five members. Similarity for RSBY is its financing mechanism which also envisages that premiums are paid by the Central and state governments in the proportion of 75:25. It is targeted at Below Poverty Line (BPL) families and has been implemented in 15 States. RSBY extends coverage through public and private hospitals and also pays transportation charges between Rs. 100–1000.

The merit of RSBY is that it works across India even though an individual signs in a chosen district, since enrolment data is disseminated across the country, and this is very significant for rural population coverage. Over the years, budgetary expenditure on RSBY (which at present is Rs. 1100 crores) has grown twice in 2010–2013. In terms of enrolment under RSBY the government publications indicate[2] that across 15 Indian states including Assam, Bihar, Chhatisgarh, Gujarat, Himachal Pradesh, Karnataka, Manipur, Meghalaya, Mizoram, Nagaland, Orissa, Tripura, Uttarakhand and West Bengal, 278 districts were identified for RSBY and of them 267 have been empanelled. Also, out of 59,117,989 total BPL families in these districts, 36,332,475 BPL families have been covered. RSBY has, in these districts, empanelled 4,926 private and 3,771 public hospitals. This is an indication that RSBY has grown in desired directions and thus should be a useful precursor for the NHP.

It is observed that RSBY is extended to 80 per cent in Mizoram and the lowest at 49 per cent in Nagaland. With the largest number of BPL families, Assam in Northeastern India covered 59.91 per cent in the same scheme.[3]

RSBY covers hospitalization up to Rs. 30,000 per annum and Union Ministry of Health and Family Welfare administers it. States in this regard have their separate nodal agencies. Further, district level coverage also varies within a state. For instance, in Assam, it ranged from 18,120 to 4,458 across Nagaon and Dima Hasao districts. Nevertheless, official surveys like NFHS in 2015–2016 indicated only 10.4 per cent insurance under RSBY. Although earlier in 2005–2006, it was only 2.3 per cent.[4]

Despite increasing coverage, lack of awareness also plagues RSBY. Even after campaigns by the government, many people do not come forward to avail of the benefits of the health schemes, thus causing lower enrolment. According to the National Family Health Survey 2015–16, only 10.4 per cent population in Assam is covered by a health insurance scheme. However, in its earlier survey that took place in 2005–2006, the percentage was only 2.3.[5]

Additionally, in terms of failure of removing demerit of low coverage under RSBY, even the health ministry's proposal to raise the cover of Rs 100,000 did not work out, as many states are allowing higher claims.

In terms of duplication of efforts by different tiers of government, it is noteworthy that besides the National Health Insurance by the central fund, apart from 12 Indian states, all other states have their own health insurance schemes. The states which do not have any state level health insurance include Punjab, Haryana, Delhi, Bihar, Madhya Pradesh, Uttar Pradesh, Kerala, Nagaland and Sikkim.

The states that currently have their own state-sponsored scheme generally also cover BPL families. For instance, among the southern states, Tamil

Nadu, Andhra Pradesh and Karnataka have state-level health insurance schemes. Most of them also use the mechanism of their health insurance schemes running through a tie up with an existing health insurance company in India. Tamil Nadu state government has a tie up with the United India Insurance Company. The latter provides free medical and surgical treatment in government and private hospitals and particularly those with annual family income less than Rs. 72,000 benefit from it. The previous state insurance scheme (in Tamil Nadu), named the Kalaignar Insurance Scheme, was operational from 2009 to 2012 and was affiliated with the private Star Insurance Company for the provision of private facilities.

The existing Chief Minister's Comprehensive Health Insurance Scheme covers every member of a family in lower income bracket (below Rs. 72,000/-). This scheme is currently envisaged to cover approximately 1.34 crore (13,400,000) people. Using a smartcard encrypted with medical details, the scheme benefits to an extent of Rs. 1 lakh per annum. Even certain conditions requiring expenditure up to Rs. 1.5 lakhs are permitted. It is a completely cashless transaction up to their insurance limit. The scheme covers 1,016 procedures, 113 follow up procedures and 23 diagnostic procedures. The cost of tests required for treatment would also be part of the insurance cover. More than 250 hospitals are empanelled under the scheme. At least six hospitals in each district would be covered. There would be more hospitals in cities such as Chennai, Coimbatore and Madurai.

Likewise, in Andhra Pradesh, the state government is implementing Dr Nandamuri Taraka Rama Rao Vaidya Seva Health Insurance Scheme (Dr NTR Vaidya Seva Health Insurance Scheme). This scheme provides Universal Health Coverage to BPL families. The scheme uses a PPP model and works through networking services between government and private sectors. The scheme is designed in such a way that at the primary care level IEC activities and free screening and outpatient consultation, both in the health camps and in the network hospitals, are a part of scheme implementation. The state government manages the scheme through Dr NTR Vaidya Seva Trust, which is headed by the chief minister and run by government functionaries. It provides the choice of hospital for treatment to the patient. It has the meritorious feature that the entire process of service provisioning including screening, diagnosing, treatment, follow-up and claim payment is web based, thus preventing any misuse and fraud. The scheme complements government hospital facilities. The scheme provides coverage for the 1,044 "listed therapies" for identified diseases in the 29 categories – which are listed on the state government website:[6] The Scheme is intended to benefit 129.44 lakh families in all 13 districts of the state. It also reimburses transport charges as per the Scheme norms and obtains receipts. The Andhra scheme has expanded through PPP framework to cover journalist and advanced facilities like haemodialysis in 11 government hospitals, and other diagnostic facilities in Government Hospitals.

In Karnataka, the state government funded scheme launched in June 2018 is called Arogya Karnataka (or Karnataka Arogya Bhagya) scheme and it promises to uplift the overall medical status of the state. The main objective of this scheme is to offer health facilities for all. The motto of this Karnataka state government sponsored project is "Health for all." It is estimated that the scheme will be able to offer better and free medical assistance to around 1.4 crore legal residents of Karnataka. Under this all BPL receive free care and APL will have to pay 70 per cent of the treatment cost, while the state government will pay only 30%. The scheme will offer as much as Rs. 1.5 lakh to meet the medical expenses of each family, during every financial year. Additional monetary assistance for treatment is available – if any member of the family is suffering from serious illness, and requires more money for treatment, the state authority will offer an additional financial assistance of Rs. 50,000. This scheme allows referral to private hospitals only if government specified government hospitals do not have that treatment facility. Currently many hospitals are included in the list of empanelled hospitals and there are plans to expand this panel. Using a smart card issued under the scheme, it will allow the common people of the state to access primary, secondary and tertiary care, as well as emergency healthcare services.

Among north Indian states, in Rajasthan for instance, a state health insurance called Bhamashah Swasthya Bima Yojana has operated since 2014–2015. The scheme was initially aimed at National Food Security Scheme (NFSS) families, such that workload on government Health Institutions is reduced. Now it also covers the RSBY (Rashtriya Swasthya Bima Yojana) beneficiaries. It uses cashless treatment and aims to improve quality of care as well as efficiency. Using Bhamashah Cards or identity related to NFSS and RSBY this scheme has a coverage of Rs. 30,000/- for general illnesses and Rs. 3.00 lakhs for critical on a floater basis in one year for inpatient (IPD) procedures.

The New India Assurance Company has been contracted for the scheme. Presumably for its coverage BSBY will encourage the private sector to establish hospitals in rural areas and thus reduce the burden on government facilities. However, Rajasthan's ambitious health insurance scheme excludes many poor patients since it requires too many documents, has no checks on hospitals and takes no action on denial of treatment.

In central India, since 2013, a state-level health insurance scheme also runs in Maharashtra, called Jyotiba Phule Jan Arogya Yojana (MJPJAY). It is interesting to note that as per the state's official estimate, in contrast to envisaged central scheme coverage of 40 per cent of the state population, the existing health insurance scheme of the state already covers about 75 per cent. The MJPJAY scheme caters to 2.20 crore families or 9 crore people, with health care services of up to Rs 1.5 lakh. The state government offers 971 procedures by paying Rs 690 as premium per year per family. Its merit lies in its better and higher coverage than central schemes.

Among western states, in Gujarat, a scheme called Mukhyamantri Amrutam "MA" & "MA Vatsalya" Yojana has been operating since 2012. Meant for BPL people and lower income groups, at present it covers families with incomes of Rs. 1.50 lakh to Rs. 2.50 lakh per annum for "MA Vatsalya" beneficiaries. Recently the income limit has been increased from Rs. 2.50 lakh to Rs. 3.00 lakh per annum for MA V Strategies & Programme. All beneficiaries can avail of cashless quality medical and surgical treatment for catastrophic illnesses related to cardiac, renal and nervous system, fire injuries, malignancies, neo-natal diseases, joints and vital organs and uses a classification encompassing 698 defined procedures. The sum assured varies according to type of treatments. Additional cost is borne by the beneficiary and transportation charges for every instance of availing treatment from the empanelled hospital are paid by the scheme. To avail of benefits every family has been issued a QR coded card (Quick Response Coded Card). "MA Vatsalya" Card is compulsory for availing of treatment. IEC activities, mega health camps, media publicity, and enrolments through mobile kiosks are also carried out under the scheme. This is scheme is entirely funded by the state and the service providers are paid through it. This scheme thus overcomes the lack of awareness among people and has the merit of using information technology.

Until recently in the hilly state of Uttarakhand Mukhyamantri Swasthya Beema Yojna (MSBY), a health insurance scheme, provided cashless health benefits for its holders in case of hospitalization in public as well as private hospitals. However, the scheme has been rolled back. The scheme covered 12.5 lakh people in the state who were not taxpayers, pensioners or government employees. The insurance was available in hospitals including 94 public hospitals and 84 private hospitals. It allowed cashless cover of Rs 1.75 lakh to each family. The government sources indicated causes like contract non-renewal with existing private firms for discontinuation of the scheme. The scheme was rolled out in 2015. However, in May this year over three lakh families who had the health cover were left without insurance cover as their health cards had been deactivated.

In the northeast, Assam has a health insurance scheme called as Atal Amrit Abhiyan. Announced in 2016 it covers a sum of up to Rs. 2 Lakh per year. It is aimed at health care treatment coverage for BPL and APL families besieged with chronic, sudden or acute health issues. It also covers treatment for critical and dread disease. People suffering from these diseases would be able to get treatment at all government and CGHS empanelled hospitals for up to Rs. 2 Lakh. The scheme works through smart card and is free for the BPL families. 437 diseases would be covered under Atal Amrit Abhiyan which has been segregated in six groups. According to official estimate, it may cover nearly 90 per cent of the state's population. The state government would bear an additional burden of Rs. 200 crores to implement the scheme in the state. The government is also aiming to empanel more hospitals under the scheme.

Despite the promise of coverage by government health insurance, it does not always guarantee that the burden of treatment is being borne by the state-run schemes. Reports and criticism indicate that many times households covered by government-funded health insurance have to use personal funds to pay for hospitalization.[7] A study found that 66 per cent in public hospitals and 95 per cent in private hospitals had to pay for treatment, despite being insured with a state-sponsored coverage (Nandi, Schneider and Dixit, 2017).

Yet at the moment, Rashtriya Swasthya Bima Yojana and other state-funded health insurance schemes cover over 200 million people, while private insurance plans take the total number of insured people in India to about 360 million - about 30 per cent of the population.

But this coverage is also not always free from problems. For instance, a recent study by Public Health Resource Network,[8] a non-government entity, analysed health spending for hospitalization by insured households in Chhattisgarh. Notably the state has one of the highest enrolment population rates in government-financed health insurance. It is observed by the study that schemes typically pay from Rs 30,000 to Rs 100,000 for certain hospital-based services and yet expressed concern about plans to expand government financed health insurance. It is found that households under the scheme in Chhattisgarh should have received fully cashless services for specified conditions but only 34 per cent of hospitalization episodes in public hospitals and only five per cent in private hospitals were actually cashless services. Generally, empanelled hospitals do not follow package rates and the government is unable to regulate or enforce the contract.

Ayushman Bharat (or MODI CARE) / PMJAY (Prime Minister's Jan Arogya Yojana)

Within this context of coverage, merits, demerits and gaps in the existing state insurance interventions discussed above, the new initiative by the central government, enunciated in the 2018 budget speech, emphasized that "India cannot realize its demographic dividend without its citizens being healthy." Moreover, with that another health insurance scheme was announced. Called Ayushman Bharat to cover over 10 crore poor and vulnerable families (approximately 50 crore beneficiaries) providing coverage up to 5 lakh rupees per family per year for secondary and tertiary care hospitalization. This is claimed to be world's largest government funded health care programme. Fondly designated as MODI Care, this scheme aims to increase the insurance cover by over 1500 per cent from Rs. 30,000 under the existing Rashtriya Swasthya Bima Yojana (RSBY), to Rs.5 lakhs.

The scheme aims to cover 100 million families (or 500 million individuals) from financially vulnerable households, enumerated under socio economic caste census (SECC) 2011 of Indian census. According to latest Census in

India, 41.3 per cent of the population falls under this. Thus, it implies that within its ambit, the NHP would cover four in ten Indians and therefore they may utilize health care in government and private hospitals, using the insurance amount earmarked per family. In line with other government schemes, Aadhar biometric is going be the base for valid identity to register under NHP. Initial approval by cabinet had set a premium of Rs. 2000 per month for each beneficiary family. However, the recent announcements from the government suggest that beneficiaries will not have to pay any premium as it will be covered by state and central government in the ratio of 40 and 60 per cent. For this cashless treatment scheme the taxpayer will pay 1 per cent extra as a health cess. An estimated 11000 crores might be collected by the cess and thus a sum of 10,000 to 20,000 crores will be allocated in the central budget outlay annually. At present the first stage will be funded by total 10,000 crores, shared between states and centre in a 40 and 60 per cent ratio. The central government has already launched this scheme in October 2018. The scheme now also has a mission director from the central government.

MODI care or PMJAY: An Approach towards Universal Health Care: Merits and Demerits

There is no doubt that the scheme has a potential to serve the nation and the nation's poor. It has all the plusses. It is interesting to note that a review of relevant literature indicates that universal health coverage in other developed or industrialized countries was made possible through financing from cess or tax specifically levied for health care. Initially in Europe many nations could make universal health coverage possible for artisans and farmers and worker class through the financing mechanism of a tax or a cess, and it survives there now as we see today. Excepting America, which did not initially aim at a government subsidized care, most other countries could provide health coverage to the needy as an affordable commodity through such financing mechanisms. The scheme is set in the context of a growing insurance business in India and Modi's mantra to develop market mechanisms which could survive in the times to come. Like the earlier RSBY, Ayushman Bharat has already started empanelling hospitals, called Health and Wellness centres. It is expected that nearly 1.5 lakh centres will be established across the country. These centres in turn will be getting their funding from the government budgets. As such, the scheme is termed as Ayushman Bharat due to its key features of National Health Protection (NHP) and Health and Wellness centres. The latter are meant for the provision of non-communicable diseases, provision of post-natal care and distribution of medicines and diagnostics. Also many studies[9] in India, particularly in Andhra Pradesh and Kerala, suggest that the existing Rashtriya Swasthya Bima Yojana (RSBY), developed on similar lines, has been fairly successful in creating new hope for affordable universal coverage.

Secondly, given the implementation mechanism of NHP, the experience of RSBY should be a useful input in its potential success. Thirdly, the NHP will go a long way in increasing expenditure on health care in India. This can be foreseen in the supply and demand factors envisaged under the scheme. For instance, for greater accessibility to healthcare, more Government Medical Colleges and Hospitals are planned to be instituted, such that there is at least one medical college for every three parliamentary constituencies. At present, there are 479 medical colleges affiliated to the Medical Council of India (MCI) whereas we have 543 parliamentary constituencies. Presently spatial distribution is uneven, and more colleges are clustered around urban centres. At present, the country has a density of one medical college per 38.41 lakh population and there are 315 medical colleges that are located in 188 of 642 districts. As predicted by a high-level expert group on Universal Health Coverage at erstwhile Planning Commission, this situation would take at least 17 years to reach the World Health Organization's norm of one doctor per 1000 people.[10] A World Health Organization report (WHO, 2017) on the Health Workforce in India states that on an average, there are 64.9 physicians per one lakh people in the country.[11] Currently, Chandigarh tops with the highest doctors per capita (279.9 doctors per lakh population). Meghalaya is a contrast to this, with 27.5 doctors per lakh. Mostly the north-eastern states are lower than the national average in terms of overall healthcare manpower. For instance, Arunachal Pradesh and Nagaland also have 32.5 and 35.6 doctors per lakh respectively. With the demand for health care rising, and with the potential success of MODI Care, it is very likely that medical manpower average per capita will increase. Further, there is a likelihood that the present health expenditure per capita estimated to be US$267 in 2014, which happens to be much lower than world average of US$1,271, may in due course increase. Following the World Bank data, India's per capita spending is even lower than other developing countries like Indonesia, and the African nations of Djibouti and Gabon, with their average citizen spending US$338 and US$599 respectively on healthcare. In fact, some study reports suggest developed countries view health as an investment to promote more economically equitable society. This is an overall good bargain to initiate measures for increasing per capita health expenditure in the country.

So far, 20 states have signed memorandums of understanding with the centre to implement the National Health Protection Scheme (NHP). West Bengal, Kerala, Tamil Nadu and Delhi are some of the states that have not signed up yet. West Bengal had shown interest but has not sent any formal request, it was revealed at the health ministers' conclave on the NHP. Twelve states have decided to take the insurance route for payments to hospitals. These include Uttarakhand, Haryana, Nagaland, Tripura and Meghalaya. Gujarat, Kerala, Himachal Pradesh and Tamil Nadu which have decided to adopt the hybrid model, where part of the payment will be made through insurance and the rest through trusts. In Gujarat, payments may also be made through trusts for claims above Rs 50,000.

Among the states that are adopting this scheme, Uttar Pradesh, Haryana and Bihar do not have their own health insurance schemes and constitute 30–40 per cent of the total beneficiaries. Telangana, Andhra Pradesh and Rajasthan have their own schemes but are going with the NHPS. A pilot project in Haryana has actually revealed that socio-economic Caste Census (SECC) data was successful in tracing 80 per cent of families in target villages.

Another important point to consider is the fact that MODI Care aims to replace state-sponsored health insurance schemes, presumably to bring uniformity across the states, yet it may discourage the efforts that should constitutionally be performed by them. This in turn would mean shifting the onus of taxation from states to central government to bear this additional burden. The implied consequence is the further weakening of state efforts to increase their finance raising ability and an overall downward trend for welfare measures at the state level. This may be an additional step to deepen the vertical fiscal imbalance between centre and states.

On the flip side, bringing uniformity across the implementation of health insurance through MODI Care may also be hailed as a good measure. Nonetheless, it takes away some state-level uniqueness in formulation and implementation of health schemes. Now each state-level, state-run health insurance has a uniqueness of architecture suited to the social and economic fabric in the respective states. Thus, this angle of losing state-level uniqueness and the weakening of political benefit that the ruling parties have in the states currently due to their respective health schemes could be an impediment for its smooth implementation.

Thirdly, the continuation of MODI Care at the cost of coverage states like Maharashtra face may also be an important consideration to reckon with. As the reports suggest, the present state-sponsored health insurance in Maharashtra already covers more of the population relative to proposed MODI Care implementation, thus it is an obvious disadvantage for this particular state.

Finally, it should also be mentioned that comparing MODI Care to Obamacare is indeed impressive, yet it is more of a dubious comparison. It is noteworthy that there are sheer differences in context, coverage and size between the two. As per Obama estimates, it was stated to be US$940 billion in the next 10 years, whereas the American Congressional Budget Office came out with an estimated cost of US$1.76 trillion. In India, the cost is lower and much less. In India, the scheme is specifically targeted at India's poor while Obamacare was for the poor but also benefited middle class Americans. In America, it is mandatory to buy insurance cover, for which Obamacare offered government subsidy on the premiums. In India, it might cover and benefit a larger population at a lower cost with nearly the entire premium paid by the government. In comparison to MODI Care's

Rs 5 lakh limit, Obamacare has no such limit or cap for essential health benefits. The US Affordable Care Act ensures that in the case of chronic illness, policyholders get health cover even if they have run out of coverage. Lastly, India is a low health spender in terms of GDP, which is estimated to be 1.15 per cent of GDP, and it is expected to be 2.5 per cent of the GDP by 2025. By contrast, the United States spends around 18 per cent of its GDP on healthcare, thus making a comparison with such a contextual difference unwarranted.

Conclusions and Policy Imperatives

Overall, taking into consideration various aspects of our health systems, literature review and the merits and demerits of existing arrangements of other state interventions in health insurances, it may require a more cautious approach to implement MODI Care throughout the nation. Appreciably, it can go a long way in mitigating inequality in healthcare across the country. However, merging all the state-level insurance schemes under the new cover may be like throwing the baby with the bathwater. In addition, we must give utmost importance to the available infrastructure that is in many states and rural areas nearly non-existent or nonfunctioning. Though NRHM has helped, much more effort is required to make these health facilities more useful and fully functional.[12] The government has to fasten the speed of availability of doctors, nurses, wellness centres and hospitals. Secondly, while involving private insurance policy providers some norms have to be fixed and some centralized agency governing these providers should be roped in. Thirdly, and more importantly, we need to have a centralized as well as state wise decentralized mechanism to govern the implementation of this scheme. To be sure, this department should not be adorned by only babujis (clerks). It must have health specialists, health managers and doctors as well as senior officials. Fourthly, many studies have observed that empanelment of private hospitals is more relative to public hospitals in these types of state-sponsored schemes in India and the charges fixed for reimbursement for these hospitals are not covering many items, thus burdening the insured to pay out of pocket expenses which are otherwise avoidable with proper rate fixing. Finally, the general notion of quality and availability of healthcare facilities being better at private hospitals and the nearer availability of such facilities relative to public hospitals also prompts the seekers to go for private health facility utilization and end up with more out of pocket expenses despite the good intention of state-sponsored health insurance schemes. Thus, besides usual components of state-run health insurance (like MODI Care) reimbursing to private providers, some thinking and policy is needed to pep up and upgrade public hospitals and facilities to gain an increased credibility for the healthcare seekers in the country, to smoothen the implementation and achieve the desired outcome of an effective universal coverage.

Notes

1 See Appendix Tables adopted from above reference of Shekhar, 2016
2 http://www.rsby.gov.in/overview.aspx; last viewed 2nd August 2018.
3 http://www.rsby.gov.in/statewise.aspx?state=16; last viewed 2nd August 2018.
4 http://www.rsby.gov.in/statewise.aspx?state=16; last viewed 2nd August 2018.
5 International Institute for Population Sciences (IIPS) and ICF. 2017. National Family Health Survey (NFHS-4), India, 2015-16: Assam. Mumbai: IIPS.
6 See, www.ntrvaidyaseva.ap.gov.in
7 Nandi S, Schneider H, Dixit P (2017) Hospital utilization and out of pocket expenditure in public and private sectors under the universal government health insurance scheme in Chhattisgarh State, India: Lessons for universal health coverage. PLoS ONE 12(11): e0187904. https://doi.org/10.1371/journal.pone.0187904
8 See endnote ix above.
9 Prinja S, Chauhan AS, Karan A, Kaur G, Kumar R (2017) Impact of Publicly Financed Health Insurance Schemes on Healthcare Utilization and Financial Risk Protection in India: A Systematic Review. PLoS ONE 12(2): e0170996. doi:10.1371/ journal.pone.0170996
    Jisha C.J. (2013)The Comprehensive Health Insurance Scheme in Kerala (CHIS): An Exploratory Study in Kollam
    District, Proceedings of International Conference on Global Public Health and Social Work ISBN 978-93-82338-40-6 l; Bonfring
10 High Level Expert Group Report on Universal Health Coverage for India Instituted by Planning Commission of India, Submitted to the Planning Commission of India, New Delhi November, 2011
11 WHO (2017), World Health Statistics 2017: Monitoring health for the SDGs, Geneva
12 Purohit Brijesh C. (2014), Efficiency of Social Sector Expenditure in India, Routledge/ Francis and Taylor, UK.;Purohit Brijesh C, Health Care System Efficiency: A Sub-State Level Analysis For Orissa (India), Review of Urban and Regional Development Studies, John Wiley and Sons Australia, March 2016, pp. 1–20.

References

Ahlin, Tanja, Mark Nichter, and Gopukrishnan Pillai (2016). "Health insurance in India: What do we know and why is ethnographic research needed." *Anthropology & Medicine* 23(1): 102–124. DOI: 10.1080/13648470.2015.1135787

Barai-Jaitly, Tejal and Soumitra Ghosh (June 23, 2018). "Role of government in funded health insurance schemes." *Economic & Political Weekly EPW* LIII(25): 21–23.

Chauhan, Tarun (2017). "A study to assess the awareness level about government recognized health insurance schemes among the urban unorganized sector in East Delhi." *Imperial Journal of Interdisciplinary Research (IJIR)* 3(8). http://www.onlinejournal.in.

Choudhury, Mita and R. Srinivasan (2011). "A study on insurance schemes of Government of India (Final Report)." March, National Institute of Public Finance and Policy, New Delhi.

Forgia, Gerard La and Somil Nagpal (2012). "Government-sponsored health insurance in India are you covered?" *Directions in Development, Human Development, 72238,* International Bank for Reconstruction and Development/The World Bank, Washington DC. www.worldbank.org.

Garg Charu, C. (2014). "Barriers to and inequities in coverage and financing of health of the informal workers in India." In *India Infrastructure Report 2013|14, The Road to Universal Health Coverage*, September 24, IDFC Institute, Bandra West Mumbai, India, pp. 236–250.

International Institute for Population Sciences (IIPS) and ICF (2017). *National Family Health Survey (NFHS-4), India, 2015–16: Assam*. Mumbai: IIPS.

Jain, Kalpana (2013). "Health financing and delivery in India: An overview of selected schemes." Women in Informal Employment: Globalizing and Organizing (WIEGO), Cambridge, MA, USA, June.

Jisha, C. J. (2013). "The Comprehensive Health Insurance Scheme in Kerala (CHIS): An exploratory study in Kollam District." Proceedings of International Conference on Global Public Health and Social Work ISBN 978-93-82338-40-6; Bonfring.

Nagaraju, Y. (2014). "A study on performance of health insurance schemes in India." *International Journal of Innovative Research and Practices* 2(4) April: 9–19.

Nandi, S., H. Schneider, and P. Dixit (2017). "Hospital utilization and out of pocket expenditure in public and private sectors under the universal government health insurance scheme in Chhattisgarh State, India: Lessons for universal health coverage." *PLoS ONE* 12(11): e0187904. DOI: 10.1371/journal.pone.0187904

Prinja, S., A. S. Chauhan, A. Karan, G. Kaur, and R. Kumar (2017). "Impact of publicly financed health insurance schemes on healthcare utilization and financial risk protection in India: A systematic review." *PLoS ONE* 12(2): e0170996. DOI: 10.1371/journal.pone.0170996

Purohit, Brijesh C. (2014). *Efficiency of Social Sector Expenditure in India*. UK: Routledge/Francis and Taylor.

Purohit, Brijesh C. (2016). "Health care system efficiency: A sub-state level analysis for Orissa (India)." *Review of Urban and Regional Development Studies*. Australia: John Wiley and Sons, pp. 1–20.

Purohit, Brijesh C. (2017). *Inequity in Indian Health Care*. Singapore: Springer Nature.

Rajasekhar, D. and R. Manjula (2012). "A comparative study of the Health insurance schemes in Karnataka." Planning Department, Government of Karnataka, December.

Rathi, A. (2017). "Health insurance a predominant medium for achieving universal healthcare in India–A farfetched dream?" *Immunology Case Reports* 1(1): 2–4.

Sarwal, Rakesh (2015). "Reforming central government health scheme into a 'Universal Health Coverage' model." *The National Medical Journal of India* 28(1): e1–e10.

Selvaraj, Sakthivel and Anup K. Karan (2012, March 17). "Why publicly-financed health insurance schemes are ineffective in providing financial risk protection." *Economic & Political Weekly* xlvii(11): 60–68.

Sharma, A., N. Oberoi, S. Singh, A. Mathur, V. P. Aggarwal, and M. Batra (2018). "Utilization of healthcare schemes: A ground reality of Indian scenario." *Journal of Oral Research and Review* 10: 45–49.

Shekhar, Vrishali (2016). *India Health Insurance Case Study, Comparison of Benefit Packages of Government Sponsored Health Insurance Programs in India*. ACCESS Health India, October.

Sood, Neeraj, Eran Bendavid, Arnab Mukherji, Zachary Wagner, Somil Nagpal, and Patrick Mullen (2014). "Government health insurance for people below poverty line in India: Quasi-experimental evaluation of insurance and health outcomes." *BMJ* 349: g5114. DOI: 10.1136/bmj.g5114 (Published 25 September).

Thomas, K. T. and R. SakthiVel (2011). "Private health insurance in India: Evaluating emerging business models." *Journal of Health Management* 13(4): 401–417.

Venkitasubramanian, Akshay (2010). "A study of PPP models for social healthcare insurance." *Working Paper Series*, Centre for Public Policy Research, December.

WHO (2017). *World Health Statistics 2017: Monitoring Health for the SDGs.* Geneva.

APPENDIX: Features of State Financed Health Insurance Schemes in India 1:(Source: Shekhar, October 2016)

State-sponsored schemes

Scheme	coverage			Annual limit	Provider network	No. of packages	opd	Target group	Extended coverage by state
	Primary	*Secondary*	*Tertiary*						
NTR Vaidya (AP)	Limited	√	√	250,000/family	Public and private	1044 with follow up	√	BPL	No
Rajiv Arogya shri (TS)	X	√	√	200,000/family	Public and private	938 and 120 follow up	×	BPL	No
Vajpayee Agyashri (KA)	X	X	√	150,000/family + 50,000 buffer	Public and private	471 packages	×	BPL	No
Rajiv Arogya Bhagya	X	×	√	150,000/family	Public and private	449 packages	×	APL	No
Chief Minister's comprehensive health insurance Scheme (TN)	X	√	√	150,000/family	Public and private	992 and 113 follow up packages	×	Annual income less than INR70,000	No
Rajiv Jeevandayi (MH)	X	√	√	150,000/family	Public and private	971 and 121 follow up packages	×	BPL and APL	No
Mukhya Mantri Amutum (GJ)	×	×	√	200,000/family	Public and private	544 packages	×	BPL and APL	No

Centrally sponsored Schemes

Scheme	Coverage			Annual limit	Provider network	No. of packages	opd	Target group	Extended coverage by state
	Primary	Secondary	Tertiary						
Rashtriya Swasthya Bima Yojana (RSBY)	x	✓	x	100,000/family and top-up for Senior citizen 30,000	Public and private	1516 and 22 daycare procedures	x	BPL population and unorganised sector	N/A
Central government health scheme (CGHS)	✓	✓	✓		Own network and private	Comprehensive	✓	Central government employees and dependents	N/A
Employees state insurance Scheme (ESIS)	✓	✓	✓		Own network and private	Comprehensive	✓	Industrial workers and dependents	N/A
Ex-serviceman contributory health scheme (ECHS)	✓	✓	✓		Own network and private	Comprehensive	✓	Ex-defence and dependents	N/A
Retired employees liberalised health scheme (RELHS)	✓	✓	✓		Own network and private	Comprehensive	✓	Railways employees and spouses	N/A

Chapter 5

Role of Public and Private Sectors in Health Insurance

As mentioned in earlier chapters, we distinguish health insurance schemes in six ways. These include government funded social security schemes, which cover health insurance like ESIS, health insurance schemes funded by the government like CGHS, central government-sponsored schemes like Ayushman Bharat or RSBY, state government-sponsored schemes including 21 state schemes mentioned in the appendix to chapter 4, community health insurance, which we discuss later in this chapter, and private health insurance purchased from the insurance companies by the individual or groups, employers and families. Among these first four categories social security schemes (including health insurance), central government funded schemes (e. CGHS) and central or state sponsored schemes are termed as public sectors schemes. The last two categories, namely private insurance and community health insurance are called private-sector health insurance schemes. It is also worth mentioning that most of the public-sector central or state sponsored schemes involve an element of public-private partnership. This element emerges through empanelling private hospitals in the provider hospital networks by the four public-sector non-life insurance companies, which are National Insurance Company Limited, New India Assurance Company Limited, Oriental Insurance Company Limited and United India Insurance Company. The hospitalisation expenses or other medical-surgical costs are reimbursed by the insurers to the hospitals directly through third party administrators. Also, we should note that other than social security health insurance schemes and government funded schemes, most of the other central or state sponsored schemes do not cover outpatient care or out of pocket expenses on account of availing healthcare under these schemes. The mechanism of reimbursement by these sponsored schemes works through public-sector insurers through Mediclaim policy (or Mediclaim mechanism). In the case of private insurance schemes, it also works through private-sector general or health insurers.

Mediclaim policy is a hospitalisation benefit that is offered by both public and private-sector general insurance companies in India. It takes care of expenses following hospitalisation/domiciliary hospitalisation in case of any

DOI: 10.4324/9781032615660-5

of the following situations including sudden illness or surgery, an accident, any surgery during the policy tenure and fees charged by medical professionals – compensation for fees charged by the doctor, surgeon, nurse, anaesthetists etc. However, every Mediclaim policy has some limitations. Some of the exclusions include coverage for: pre-existing ailments, any medical condition or critical illnesses that are diagnosed within 30 days of the policy's commencement date, some specific ailments that are not covered in the plan, expenses incurred on dental surgeries unless it requires hospitalisation, birth control and hormonal treatment and complication during childbirth and ectopic pregnancies. Due to its main focus on hospitalisation expenses and various exclusions, namely of OPD care, preventive care and other out of pocket expenses on availing health care, the Mediclaim is not considered a full-fledged health insurance. A Mediclaim plan provides coverage only for hospitalisation, accident-related treatment and pre-decided diseases for a pre-specified limit. By contrast a health insurance plan offers comprehensive coverage against hospitalisation charges, pre-hospitalisation charges, post-hospitalisation charges and ambulance expenses. It also offers compensation in case of loss of income as a result of an accident. Mediclaim doesn't offer any add-on coverage. Whereas a health insurance scheme offers critical illness coverage, personal accident coverage, accidental disability coverage, maternity coverage etc. Further, Mediclaim offers no flexibility, but a health insurance plan offers much needed flexibility. Insurance buyers can reduce their health insurance premium amount after a specified period; they can even change their policy duration. They can avail of long-term policies to enjoy maximum insurance benefits. Additionally, features of a Mediclaim plan vary from provider to provider. Generally, different (Mediclaim) insurance companies offer different Mediclaim insurance coverage. However, the benefits and features of a health insurance plan of a specific sum insured are the same over most insurance providers. Unless specified, Mediclaim does not provide coverage for critical illnesses. Whereas a health insurance would cover more than 30 plus critical diseases such as cancer, stroke, kidney failure, etc. Likewise, claim payments procedures and amounts also differ between Mediclaim and a full-fledged health insurance scheme. Lastly, Mediclaim benefits can be availed if the insured gets hospitalised, yet it is not necessary in a health insurance scheme that an insured gets hospitalised to avail of benefits like day-care procedures etc.

Based on the type of coverage, and a combination of clauses, there are currently five types of health insurance coverage in public or private-sector insurers. These are categorised under individual health plans, family floater health insurance policies,[1] senior citizen health insurance policies[2], top-up and super top-up insurance policies,[3] policies covering specific illnesses such as cancer or heart disease.[4]

Thus, as depicted in Tables 5.1–5.5, which indicate Mediclaim for instance, for one of the public-sector insurance company, namely, National Insurance

Table 5.1 Varistha Mediclaim Policy

Year	No. of policies issued	No. of persons covered	Premium received (in ')	No. of claims reported	No. of claims settled	Amount paid (in ')	Incurred claim ratio (%)
2009–2010	16333	19510	135612	2340	2177	111021	50
2010–2011	21359	25483	176134	8428	3599	100233	59.62
2011–2012	26254	31382	217311	10075	4871	142359	65.22
2012–2013	38046	45380	238347	12638	6994	171891	74.81
2013–2014	31263	37352	257641	12579	6964	214474	83.2
2014–2015	31330	37877	266596	15231	15243	257861	96
2015–2016	31255	43295	270193	14169	8113	262691	97.22
2016–2017	30773	36816	271433	11306	6667	232273	176.34
2017–2018	30526	37152	269355	10445	5940	270134	100.29

Table 5.2 Rashtriya Swasthya Bima Policy

RSBY

year	No. of policies issued	No. of persons covered	Premium received (in ')	No. of claims reported	No. of claims settled	Amount paid (in ')	Incurred claim ratio (%)
2009–2010	18	8368751	358967	18135	14355	136271	50
2010–2011	33	14111136	805357	135632	104017	580892	72.12
2011–2012	38	15496416	944100	242149	208220	1277900	54.76
2012–2013	65	11752608	2187144	149122	132534	1307774	61.79
2013-14	97	28600000	1799577	2023	1823	1713052	83.06
2014-15	107	3016607	1750092	236116	167071	2226003	114
2015–2016	45	–	1289028	1787	1632	2028899	173.53
2016–2017	44	–	1121377	46533	26621	2437901	224.32
2017–2018	53	15	1314079	296960	312342	1988636	151.33

Table 5.3 Parivar Mediclaim Policy

Year	No. of policies issued	No. of persons covered	Premium received (in ')	No. of claims reported	No. of claims settled	Amount paid (in ')	Incurred claim ratio (%)
2009–2010	82900	252958	571255	10547	9442	344025	70
2010–2011	115070	353990	810625	25620	16570	527437	66.39
2011–2012	142836	440917	1040997	32931	21872	725367	75.48
2012–2013	199175	617858	1225758	42722	31897	1009084	80.85
2013–2014	209795	654982	1410832	47185	35610	1319786	93.5
2014–2015	207644	655256	1676920	57893	56736	1540105	92
2015–2016	225785	831960	1866768	68162	52033	1896350	101.58
2016–2017	233023	724710	1992189	72584	49925	1898189	195.54
2017–2018	53439	165535	435667	17112	13224	432691	99.32

Table 5.4 Vidyarthi Mediclaim Policy

Year	No. of policies issued	No. of persons covered	Premium received (in ')	No. of claims reported	No. of claims settled	Amount paid (in ')	Incurred claim ratio (%)
2010–2011	3396	6107	23550	1377	490	11762	53.46
2011–2012	4060	6454	25280	1403	447	10024	60.98
2012–2013	3844	7741	23882	1677	727	14859	46.24
2013–2014	4041	6699	30304	1557	510	13117	43
2014–2015	4180	7946	34790	1820	1846	15430	45
2015–2016	4088	7826	32175	1432	509	16195	50.33
2016–2017	3780	6250	35521	958	400	16405	94.4
2017–2018	3609	6217	41556	798	413	17015	40.95

Table 5.5 Universal Health Insurance Scheme

Year	No. of policies issued	No. of persons covered	Premium received (in ')	No. of claims reported	No. of claims settled	Amount paid (in ')	Incurred claim ratio (%)
2009–2010	95379	320535	129701	9253	9127	110976	80
2010–2011	91511	302305	211173	16327	11161	173402	89.38
2011–2012	62642	213914	194270	17194	12205	206402	111.17
2012–2013	140900	829354	75601	11465	10557	47932	63.4
2013–2014	31583	100461	39813	11307	7602	69328	174.41
2014–2015	29103	93134	40391	8622	8850	52939	128
2015–2016	25550	80550	40933	7460	5269	49274	120
2016–2017	21732	49780	37584	7477	4899	51847	247
2017–2018	17129	34163	36166	6511	3588	45492	125.79

Company (Mediclaim), suggests that from 2010–2016, the coverage and premium for Mediclaim under different government-sponsored or funded insurance schemes has been increasing for policies including Varishtha, RSBY, Parivar, Vidyarthi and Universal Health Insurance schemes. Also, premiums and coverage for some other schemes like Gramin Suswasthya Micro Insurance Policy, National Mediclaim and National Mediclaim Plus have been increasing (see Annexure 2 Tables 5.A2.1–5.A2.3).

Using the underlying Mediclaim mechanism, many private insurance companies are also offering different health insurance schemes. As mentioned above, these cover individuals, family, senior citizens and offer coverage for dread or chronic diseases. Some of the major private insurance companies in India offering one or more of these types of products include Bajaj Allianz, Bharti Axa, Cholamandalam, Future Generali, HDFC Ergo, ICICI Lombard, IffcoTokio, L&T General, RahejaQbe, Reliance, Royal Sundaram, SBI General Shriram, Tata AIG and Universal Sompo.

Further, IRDA, as on March 31, 2012, has granted licenses to three insurance companies to operate as stand-alone health insurance companies, exclusively in the health insurance segments. The names of these insurers are Star Health and Allied Insurance Co Ltd., Apollo Munich Health Insurance Co Ltd. and Max Bupa Health Insurance Co Ltd. These insurance companies are authorised to underwrite business in health, personal accident and travel insurance segments. Further, IRDA has granted license to the Religare Health Insurance Co. Ltd., a new stand-alone health insurer in the year viz. 2012–2013. The performance of these companies in initial years is given in Annexure 1 below. Some of the major health insurance plans by these private insurers are briefly given in Annexure 1, Table 5.A1.1. Also, the new health insurance plans by the private insurers cleared by IRDA are mentioned in Annexure 1, Table 5.A1.2.

Public and Private Sectors Insurers in India: Some Financial Parameters

The growth in premiums collected by the public, private and private stand-alone health insurers for the period 2010–2017 is shown in Figure 5.1. It indicates that private-sector insurers are growing faster than their public counterparts. However, stand-alone private health insurers are not growing as fast as others.

A similar situation in regard to the net profits of this set of insurers is depicted in Figure 5.2 which also indicates private-sector profits growing much faster than others.

Another way of looking at the health insurance business is to observe the percentage of different types of insurance, namely individual, group or

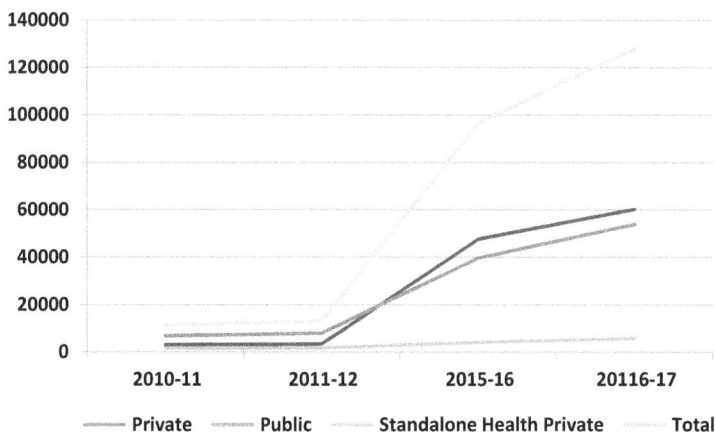

Figure 5.1 Health Insurance Premium: Public, Private and Stand-alone companies (Rs. crore) (2010–2017).

Source: Annexure 3; Table 5.A3.1.

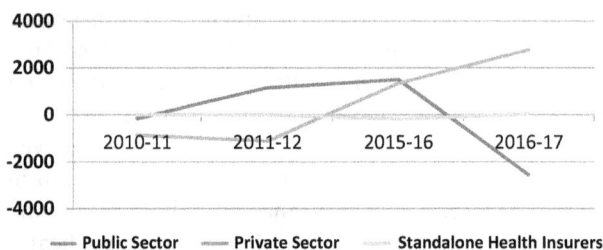

	4000				
	2000				
	0				
		2010-11	2011-12	2015-16	2016-17
	-2000				
	-4000				

— Public Sector   — Private Sector   — Standalone Health Insurers

Figure 5.2 Health Insurers' Net profits: Public, Private and Stand-alone companies (Rs. crore) (2010--2017).

Source: Annexure 3; Table 5.A3.2.

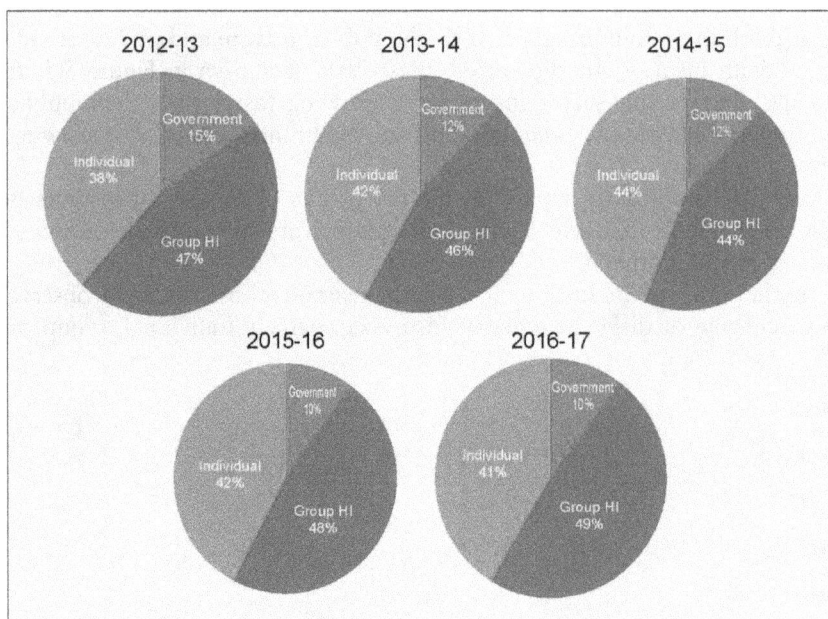

Figure 5.3 Classification of Health Insurance Business.

Source: IRDAI Annual Reports

government-sponsored insurance across all companies. This is presented in Figure 5.3. It shows that until 2015 individual insurance grew more and was 44 per cent of the total health insurance business in India. Thereafter group insurance picked up and was the highest at 49 per cent in 2016–2017. However, the government-sponsored insurance declined relative to other classes and it remained at only 10 per cent of total health insurance business in the country.

Despite this trend of growing health insurance business in the group insurance segment, the overall number of persons covered are in government-sponsored schemes (77 per cent). By contrast, the group and individual insurance coverage is only 16 and 7 per cent, respectively (Table 5.6). Yet the trend of change to group insurance business is depicted in the premium percentages, which reinforces that that share of government-sponsored schemes was higher.

Further, if we look at the efficiency of health insurance business in India, we find that it is the lowest, with claims ratios exceeding 100 per cent in public-sector companies. It is better in private-sector companies and stand-alone health insurers at around 84 and 58 per cent (Table 5.7). If we look in terms of schemes, we observe that it is exceeding 100 per cent both in government-sponsored and group schemes. It is, however, 76 per cent in individual health insurance (Table 5.8). These trends in claims ratios depict that public-sector insurance companies do subsidise health insurance through budgetary support. Also, it suggests that both the government-sponsored schemes and group insurance in health are not profitable for health insurance companies in India.[5]

Table 5.6 Number of Persons Covered under Health Insurance (Excluding Pa & Travel Insurance Business)

Class of business	2012–2013	2013–2014	2014–2015	2015–2016	2016–2017
Government-sponsored schemes including RSBY	1494	1553	2143	2733	3350
Percent to total	72%	72%	74%	76%	77%
Group business (other than govt. Business)	343	337	483	570	705
Percent to total	17%	15%	17%	16%	16%
Individual business	236	272	254	287	320
Percent to total	11%	13%	9%	8%	7%
Grand total	2073	2162	2880	3590	4375

Source: IRDAI Annual Reports.

Table 5.7 Claims Ratios across Sectors

Sector-Wise Net Incurred Claims Ratio of Health Insurers					
	2012–2013	2013–2014	2014–2015	2015–2016	2016–2017
Public-sector general insurers	103%	106%	112%	117%	122%
Private-sector general insurers	78%	87%	84%	81%	84%
Stand-alone health insurers	61%	67%	63%	58%	58%
Industry average	94%	97%	101%	102%	106%

Table 5.8 Claims Ratios across Types of Business

Class of business	2012–2013	2013–2014	2014–2015	2015–2016	2016–2017
Government-sponsored schemes including RSBY	87%	93%	108%	109%	122%
Group business (other than govt. business)	104%	110%	116%	120%	125%
Individual business	83%	83%	81%	77%	76%
Total business	94%	97%	101%	102%	106%

Community Health Financing and Health Insurance

As mentioned in chapter 3, out of total expenditure of Rs. 22013 crores on private health insurance in India in 2015–2016, community financing-based health insurance is only Rs. 39 crores (or only 0.18 per cent). According to ILO, community-based health insurance (CBHI) is a mechanism that allows for the pooling of resources to cover the costs of future, unpredictable, health-related events. It offers individuals and households protection against the uncertain risk of catastrophic medical expenses in exchange for regular payment of premiums. In this type of insurance, the targeted community is involved in defining the contribution level and collecting mechanisms, the content of the benefit package, and/or the allocation of the scheme's financial resources.[6] The report of the WHO Commission on Macroeconomics and Health, for instance, highlighted its importance by recommending that "out-of-pocket expenditures by poor communities should increasingly be channelled into 'community financing' schemes to help cover the costs of community-based health delivery.... Community financing schemes are no panacea, and have often failed, but for many places they are a promising and flexible mechanism that can often be harnessed for local needs."[7] However, many studies have raised questions about the efficacy of this mechanism of financing health care insurance.[8] Doubts have been raised about sustainability, the coverage of poor people and the types of care and impact on health care utilisation levels. However, we should mention that the scope of NGO sector is constrained by its overall size in India. For instance, if we look at the total percentage of non-profit organisations, which according to CSO data are engaged in health is only 3 per cent (Table 5.9). Of these only 4.8 per cent are involved in insurance activities. This kind of distribution of NGOs indeed suggests a lesser existing or possible scope of private community sector in health insurance.

Case Studies of Community Financing of Health Insurance

There have been case studies of different NGOs' health insurance schemes across the country. In the following three tables we present a review of

Table 5.9 Per cent of NGOs in Health Sector

State	Health
Andhra Pradesh	4
Assam	4.2
Bihar	13.3
Chhattisgarh	7.4
Delhi	4
Gujarat	4.2
Haryana	1
Karnataka	1.4
Kerala	1.3
Madhya Pradesh	5.9
Maharashtra	6.3
Manipur	3.8
Orissa	1.9
Punjab	3.9
Rajasthan	10.2
Tamil Nadu	5.1
Uttar Pradesh	0.8
Uttarakhand	2.6
West Bengal	3.9
India	3

Source: CSO (2012); adapted from Das and Rajeev Kumar (2016).

various schemes, based on three studies. These include studies by Dhingra (2001), Ranson (2003) and Panda et al. (2014). These studies respectively cover 17, 8 and 3 community financed health insurance across different geographical regions. Thus, considering these 28 schemes as a snapshot of the existing community financed health insurance sector, we aim at having an idea of the scope of this segment of private-sector insurance in India.

Table 5.10 below is derived from Dhingra (2001) which provides two aspects, population coverage and the coverage of inpatient or outpatient care, pertaining to 16 community financed health insurance schemes.

As is observed in Table 5.10, the population coverage varies between 450 to two lakh in these schemes. Likewise, except for Aga Khan Health services, all other schemes provide only direct delivery of inpatient care.

Table 5.11 provides an overview of these two aspects for eight schemes with three of them, namely, ACCORD, SEBA and SEWA also mentioned in the Table 5.10. The observation from Table 5.11 also indicates that target population, or enrolled population in these schemes varies from 13,000 to 8 lakh with coverage of inpatient care only. It is also noteworthy from Table 5.11 that there are three schemes namely ACCORD, SEBA and SEWA that have a partnership through GIC with Mediclaim's underlying

Table 5.10 Coverage of Population and Inpatient/Outpatient Care (Pertaining to 16 Community Financed Health Insurance Schemes)

Name, location and year of initiation	Size of enrolled population	Benefits (direct vs indirect)
1. Aga Khan Health Services (AKHS), Sidhpur, Gujarat (Meloj Milk Cooperative) (1996)	450	Benefits include free outpatient consultation, discounted drugs and direct delivery. Diagnostic services.
2. Action for Community Organization Rehabilitation and Development (ACCORD), Nilgiris, Tamil Nadu (1991)	7000	Direct delivery
3. Apollo Hospital Association Madras, Tamil Nadu (1986)	10000	Direct delivery
4. Breach Candy Hospital, Bombay.	Corporate clients	
5. Goalpara, Shantiniketan, Rural West Bengal (1984)	1247	
6. Mallur Milk Cooperative, Karnataka (1973)	7000	Direct delivery
7. Medinova Health Card Scheme, Calcutta.	35000	Direct delivery
8. Raigarh, Ambikapur Health Association, Raigarh, Orissa (1974)	75000	Direct Delivery
9. Saheed Shibsankar Sabha Samiti (SSSS) Burdwan, West Bengal (1978).	6800	Direct delivery
10. Seba Cooperative Health Society (with GIC), Calcutta, West Bengal (1982)	<3000 families	Direct delivery
11. Self-Employed Women's Association (with GIC)Ahmedabad, Gujarat (1992)	15000	Direct delivery
12. Sewagram Kasturba Hospital, Wardha, Maharashtra (1972)	14390	Direct delivery
13. Social Work and Research Centre (SWRC), Ajmer, Rajasthan (1972)	20000	Direct delivery
14. Students Health Home, Calcutta, West Bengal (1955)	1,020000	Direct delivery
15. Tribhuvandas Foundation, Anand, Rural Gujarat (1993-94)	16 to 20 per cent of the target population of 800000	Indirect delivery
16. Voluntary Health Services (VHS), Medical Aid Plan, Chennai, Tamil Nadu (1963)	124715	Direct delivery

Source: derived from Reeta Dhingra (2001), NGOs and Health Insurance Schemes In India, Health and Population- Perspectives and Issues 24(4): 206-217.

Table 5.11 Inventory of Non-Governmental, Non-profit Health Insurers (Schemes Covering Inpatient Care Only) in India

Name, location, year of initiation, nature of scheme and ownership/management	Target population, type of membership, size of enrolled population	Benefits
ACCORD Nilgiris, Tamil Nadu Established 1991 NGO-intermediated (with GIC as insurer)	Adivasis 6 months–70 years of age Voluntary Individual 4446 out of13000	All hospitalisations to a maximum of Rs 1500 Covers care at one trust hospital (or others if referral required)
KKVS Madurai, Tamil Nadu Established 2000 NGO- owned	Women members of self-help groups (SHG) and their families, age 12 months–55 years. Excludes those with a history of chronic disease Voluntary Family or individual 5710 out of a general population of 69 278	Reimbursement of 75% of hospital expenses up to Rs 10 000 per family per year Except in an emergency, benefit only for treatment at Kadamalaikkundu Hospital
Navsarjan Trust Patan, Gujarat Established 1999, discontinued 2000 NGO- intermediated (with GIC as insurer)	Dalits (scheduled caste), 5–80 years of age Voluntary Individual 574 individuals	Hospitalisations to a maximum of Rs 15 000
Seba Calcutta, West Bengal Established 1982NGO- intermediated (with GIC as insurer)	Information on characteristics of target population: na Voluntary Family <3000 families	Hospitalisation expenses up to Rs 8000

(Continued)

Table 5.11 (Continued)

Name, location, year of initiation, nature of scheme and ownership/management	Target population, type of membership, size of enrolled population	Benefits
SEWA Ahmedabad, Gujarat Established 1992 NGO-intermediated (with GIC as insurer)	Self-employed women and their spouses (ages 19–58 years) Voluntary Individual 92 000 of 285 000in target population (2001–02)	Inpatient costs (private or public hospital) to Rs 2000Fixed deposit members receive one-time flat payment for maternity care, dentures and hearing aid
TF-old Anand, Gujarat Established 1993–94, discontinued 1999 NGO- owned	Residents of one rural district Voluntary Household 16%–20% of the target population of 800000	Discounts on inpatient care (inversely proportionate to their wealth) at a single trust hospital in the district
TF-new (Sardar Patel Insurance Scheme) Anand, Gujarat Established 2001 NGO-owned	Members of dairy co- operative, depositing at least 300 L/year Mandatory Household 113883 households (size of target population: na)	Covers 100% of direct costs of hospitalisation at any of 8 trusts hospitals but DOES NOT cover medicines
WWF Chennai, Tamil Nadu Established 2001–02 NGO-intermediated (with Royal Sundaram as insurer)	Women members of WWF and their families Voluntary Individual Data not available on enrolled population	Inpatient expenses up to Rs 7000 per year (maximum Rs 5000 per claim) Limits maternity care Rs 3000 cataract Rs 2000 bed charges Rs 100 per day

na: not available. ACCORD Action for Community Organization, Rehabilitation and Development KKVS Kadamalai Kalanjia Vattara Sangam GIC Government Insurance Company SEWA Self-Employed Women's Association TF Tribhuvandas Foundation WWF Working Women's Forum

Source: Ranson M. Kent (2003), Community-based health insurance schemes in India: A review, National Medical Journal, volume 16 number 2 March/April, pp.1–17.

Table 5.12 Community Health Insurance in Three Districts of Uttar Pradesh

District	Pratapgarh	Kanpur Dehat	Vaishali
Indicators/Scheme name	Sanjivani	Jeevan Sanjivani	Swastha Kamal
Enrolment indicators			
Households offered insurance	433	378	524
At least one member of household is enrolled	174	109	242
Enrolment rate for households (%)	40	29	46
Individuals offered insurance	2594	2264	2864
Individuals enrolled	604	334	868
Enrolment rate for individuals (%)	23	15	30
Annual CBHI premium per person/per year (Rs)	176	192	197
Coverage for hospitalisation			
Fees (cap per person per event, Rs)	6000	3000	–
Wage loss (per day, Rs) a	100	75	100
Transport (maximum coverage per episode, Rs)	100	100	–
Coverage for outpatient care			
Fees (Rs)	–	Unlimited	Unlimited
Lab tests (per year, Rs)	–	–	200
Imaging tests (per year, Rs)	–	–	300
Coverage for maternity care		–	
Caesarean (per episode, Rs)	5000	–	–

Source: Adapted from Pradeep Panda, Arpita Chakraborty, David M Dror and Arjun S Bedi (2014), Enrolment in community-based health insurance schemes in rural Bihar and Uttar Pradesh, India, *Health Policy and Planning*; 29:960-974. doi:10.1093/heapol/czt077

mechanism for reimbursement of amount spent on inpatient care by the beneficiaries enrolled in these schemes. A similar arrangement is also noted for WWF having a partnership with a private-sector insurer, namely, Royal Sundaram.

Further, a view of another three NGO operated health insurance scheme, namely Sanjivini, Jeevan Sanjivini and Swasth run in three districts of Uttar Pradesh state known as Pratapgarh, Kanpur Dehat and Vaishali is presented in Table 5.12. It can be observed from the table that the target population in these districts varies from 2264 to 2864. Also, there does not seem to be outpatient care coverage or any insurance company tie up arrangement in these schemes. Besides these case studies, we also present another two case studies of BASIX and Karuna Trust in Annexure 4 to this chapter.

Thus, these case studies apparently suggest a restricted scope for community health financing in India. Yet the merit of this mechanism for health insurance cannot be neglected. This provides a supplement to public or private-sector health insurance companies to enhance overall coverage with the reach extending to a poor, remote and vulnerable population in rural or urban areas of the country.

Annexure 1

a) Some of the Health Insurance Products by Private Insurance Companies in India

    Apollo Munich Optima Restore
    Religare NCB Super Premium
    Star Family Health Optima
    Max Bupa Health Companion Individual
    Cigna TTK Prohealth Plus
    HDFC ERGO Health Suraksha Gold Regain
    Royal Sundaram Lifeline Supreme
    Aditya Birla Active Assure Diamond
    Senior Citizen Red Carpet Health Insurance Policy
    Universal Sompo Health Insurance

c) Performance of Standalone Health insurers in their initial years in India (2010–2012)

Star Health and Allied Insurance

Star Health was the first company granted registration to underwrite business in Health, Personal Accident and Travel insurance segments in 2006–2007. In its sixth year of operations, the insurer underwrote gross direct premium of Rs. 1,085 crore in 2011–2012, which declined to 11.64 per cent as against Rs. 1,228 crore in 2010–2011. On net basis, the insurer earned net premium to the tune of Rs. 809 crore as against Rs. 831 crore in the previous year. The insurer reported underwriting loss of Rs.173 crore for 2011–2012 (underwriting loss of Rs. 8.68 crore in 2010–2011). In the year 2011–2012, the insurer reported a net loss of Rs.148 crore as against net profit of Rs. 7.39 crore in 2010–2011. The net incurred claims ratio in 2011–2012 increased to 95.76 per cent from 91.19 per cent in the previous year.

Apollo Munich Health Insurance

Apollo Munich was the second company to receive license to underwrite insurance business exclusively in the Health, Personal Accident and Travel insurance segments. In its fifth year of operations, the company underwrote gross direct premium of Rs. 476 crore in 2011–2012 as against Rs.283 crore in 2010–2011, i.e., a growth of 68.19 per cent. The earned net premium underwritten by the company stood at Rs. 301 crore in 2011–2012 as against Rs. 149 crore in 2010-11. The insurer reported underwriting loss of `77 crore in 2011–2012 (underwriting a loss of 94 crore in 2010–2011) and incurred net loss of 48 crore in 2011–2012 (net loss of 79 crore in 2010–2011). The net incurred claims ratio decreased to 58.20 per cent in 2011–2012 from 61.96 per cent in 2010–2011.

Max Bupa Health Insurance

Max Bupa is the third insurer in the Health segment and was issued certificate of registration in the year 2009–2010. The company underwrote gross direct premium of Rs. 99 crore in 2011–2012 against Rs. 25 crore in 2010–2011. The earned net premium underwritten by the company stood at Rs.51 crore in 2011–2012 as against Rs. 8 crore in 2010–2011. The underwriting loss has gone up to Rs.133 crore in 2011–2012 compared to Rs. 124 crore in 2010–2011. The insurer reported a net loss of Rs. 119 crore for 2011–2012 as against net loss of Rs.116 crore in 2010–2011. Its incurred claims ratio increased to 56.15 per cent from 49.84 per cent in the previous year.[9]

Table 5.A1.1 Some of the Health Insurance Plans offered by Private Insurance Companies in India at a Glance

Plan name	Entry age	Sum assured	Policy renewability	Features
Apollo Munich Optima Restore	Minimum – 91st day Maximum – 65 years	Rs. 3 lakh – Rs. 50 lakh	Lifelong	Restore benefit Stay active benefit Multiplier benefit E-opinion Additional cover for critical illness
Religare NCB Super Premium	Minimum – 91 days Maximum – No age bar as such		Lifelong	Automatic recharge of sum insured Lifelong renewability No claim bonus super Everyday care benefit Domestic air Ambulance cover
Star Family Health Optima	Minimum- 16 Day Maximum-	Rs. 2 lakh, Rs. 3 lakh, Rs. 4 lakh, Rs. 5 lakh, Rs. 10 lakh, and Rs. 15 lakh		Auto recharge benefit Compassionate travel Repatriation of mortal remains Road traffic accident cover Restoration of amount insured
Max Bupa Health Companion Individual	Minimum – 90 days Maximum – Age no bar	For variant 1 – Rs. 1 lakh, Rs. 2 lakh, Rs. 3 lakh, Rs. 4 lakh, Rs. 5 lakh and Rs. 10 lakh For Variant 2 - Rs. 5 lakh Rs. 7.5 lakh, Rs. 10 lakh and Rs. 12.5 lakh. For variant 3–15 lakh, Rs. 20 lakh, Rs. 30 lakh, Rs. 50 lakh and Rs. 1 crore	Lifetime	Refill benefit Animal bite Vaccination Direct claim settlement Long-term policy benefit Hospital cash benefit
Cigna TTK ProHealth Plus	Minimum- 91 days Maximum- No limit as such	Rs. 4.5 lakh, Rs. 5.5 lakh, Rs. 7.5 lakh and Rs. 10 lakh	Lifetime	Enhanced sum insured Restoration benefit Health maintenance benefit Critical illness expert opinion Maternity expenses

Plan	Entry Age	Sum Insured	Renewability	Features
HDFC ERGO Health Suraksha Gold Regain	Minimum – No limit as such Maximum –	Rs. 3 lakh, Rs. 4 lakh, Rs. 5 lakh, Rs. 7.5 lakh and 10 lakh	Lifelong	Zero sub-limits, Maternity benefit, Regain benefit, Cumulative bonus, Coverage basis
Royal Sundaram Lifeline Supreme	For children minimum – 90 days maximum – 25 years For adults minimum – 18 years Maximum – No bar as such.	Rs. 5 lakh, 10 lakh, 15 lakh, 20 lakh and 50 lakh	Lifelong	Sum insured reload, Second opinion benefit, Emergency domestic evacuation expenses, Pre-hospitalisation and post-hospitalisation charges, Organ transplant cover
Aditya Birla Diamond				Cancer hospitalisation booster, Any room upgrade, Sum insured reload benefit, Pre-hospitalisation and post-hospitalisation coverage, Unlimited sum insured reload
Star Senior Citizen Red Carpet	Minimum – 60 Maximum – 75	Rs. 7.5 lakh and 10 lakh	Lifetime	No medical screening, Pre-existing Illness cover, Medical consultation cover, Sub-limits, Hassle-free claim settlement
Universal Sompo Privilege	Minimum – 90 days Maximum – 55 years	For Basic Plan – 1 lakh – Rs. 2 lakh. For Essential Plan – Rs. 3 lakh t Rs. 5 lakh. For Privilege Plan – Rs 6 lakh to Rs 10 lakh	Lifetime	No medical screening, Specialist consultation, Convalescence benefit, Mother & child care benefit, Restore benefit

Table 5.A1.2 Health Insurance Products Cleared during the Financial Year 2011–2012

Sl. no.	Name of the insurer	Name of the product
1	Shriram General	Overseas Travel Insurance
2	Star Health and Allied Insurance	Netplus (Old name HIV Care Policy)
		Medi Classic Insurance (Senior Citizen Red Carpet Insurance)
		Family Health Optima Insurance Policy
		Medi Classic Insurance (Senior Citizen Red Carpet Insurance)
		Family Health Optima Insurance Policy
		Mediclassic Accident Care Policy - Individual
		Family Health Optima Accident Care Policy –Individual
		Family Health Optima Insurance Policy
		Senior Citizen Red Carpet
3	Tata AIG General	Wellsurance
		MediPrime
4	United India	UniCriti Care Policy
5	Universal Sompo	Universal Saral Suraksha Bima (Micro)
		Universal Sampoorna Suraksha Bima (Micro)
		K Bank Family Care Health Policy

Source: The Insurance Regulatory and Development Authority, annual report, 2011–2012.

Annexure 2

Table 5.A2.1 Gramin Swasthya Micro Insurance

Year	No. of policies issued	No. of persons covered	Premium received (in Rs.)	No. of claims reported	No. of claims settled	Amount paid (in Rs.)	Incurred claim ratio (%)
2013–2014	9753	34,601	9453	2894	2022	18376	194.39
2014–2015	664	1510	8797	1064	776	8883	83.5
2015–2016	5585	19,695	6262	1741	1119	16,383	261.63
2016–2017	4576	12,478	3954	1648	1071	9690	409
2017–2018	3148	6300	2151	782	538	4862	226.06

Table 5.A2.2 National Mediclaim Plus

Year	No. of policies issued	No. of persons covered	Premium received (in Rs.)	No. of claims reported	No. of claims settled	Amount paid (in Rs.)	Incurred claim ratio (%)
2014–2015	2824	5420	87832	809	773	7440	13
2015–2016	5833	12,488	18,7991	2601	794	54,364	28.92
2016–2017	7664	13,427	254,729	2710	1173	79,953	65.95
2017–2018	9350	10,840	306,239	3398	2462	125,727	41.06

Table 5.A2.3 National Mediclaim Policy

Year	No. of policies issued	No. of persons covered	Premium received (in `Rs.)	No. of claims reported	No. of claims settled	Amount paid (in Rs.)	Incurred claim ratio (%)
2013–2014	1,377,311	1,825,942	24,676,782	374,713	336,199	23,266,388	94.2
2014–2015	1,094,804	2,750,745	9,201,430	239,798	240,950	7,728,178	84
2015–2016	1,084,553	3,184,273	9,601,287	252,136	224,131	8,346,350	86.92
2016–2017	1,058,349	1,685,083	9,892,648	249,415	198,409	8,070,338	163.1
2017–2018	1,033,972	1,394,395	10,076,170	258,443	172,224	8,794,048	87.28

Annexure 3

Table 5.A3.1 Health Insurance Premium: Public, Private and Stand-alone Companies (Rs. crore) (2010–2017)

Insurer	2010–2011	2011–2012	2015–2016	2016–2017
Private	3031.48	3411.89	47,690.68	60,218.36
Public	6912.55	8020.73	39,694.08	53,804.96
Stand-alone health private	1535.77	1659.78	4152.66	5857.83
Total	**11,479.8**	**13,092.4**	**96,379.37***	**128,128.34**

* The total of 2015–2016 and 2016–2017 also includes Specialised Insurers premiums of 4841.95 and 8247.19 for the respective years.
Source: IRDAI annual reports.

Table 5.A3.2 Health Insurers' Net Profits: Public, Private and Stand-alone Companies (Rs. crore) (2010–2017)

Insurer	2010–2011	2011–2012	2015–2016	2016–2017
Public sector	−161.51	1152.48	1499	−2551
Private sector	−857.43	−1120.2	1333	2763
Stand-alone health insurers	0	0	−177	27
Total	−1018.9	32.29	3238	845

Source: IRDAI annual reports.

Table 5.A3.3 Incurred Claims Ratio: Public-Sector Non-life Insurers

Insurer	Net earned premium (` lakh)							Claims incurred (net) (` lakh)							Incurred claims ratio (%)						
	Fire	Health	Marine	Motor	Others	2011-12	2010-11	Fire	Health	Marine	Motor	Others	2011-12	2010-11	Fire	Health	Marine	Motor	Others	2011-12	2010-11
NATIONAL	52606	160644	17655	298092	78356	607353	476395	43175	168816	13641	258009	47766	531407	462328	82.07	105.09	77.26	86.55	60.96	87.5	97.05
NEW INDIA	137897	197465	30253	294035	127809	787459	647332	165735	192018	27764	247928	75308	708753	652487	120.19	97.24	91.77	84.32	58.92	90.01	100.8
ORIENTAL	51432	129914	25455	184789	97717	489306	431490	51582	133585	20447	191730	48009	445353	406536	100.29	102.83	80.33	103.76	49.13	91.02	94.22
UNITED	58441	192361	26173	225562	106186	608724	464763	44188	187902	21669	228084	56850	538694	438564	75.61	97.68	82.79	101.12	53.54	88.5	94.36
TOTAL	300376	680384	99536	1002477	410068	2492842	2019980	304680	682321	83522	925751	227933	2224206	1959914	101.43	100.28	83.91	92.35	55.58	89.22	97.03

Source: IRDAI annual reports.

Table 5.A3.4 Incurred Claims Ratio: Private Sector Non-life Insurers

Insurer	Net earned premium (` lakh)							Claims incurred (net) (` lakh)							Incurred claims ratio (per cent)						
	Fire	Marine	Motor	Health	Others	2011-12	2010-11	Fire	Marine	Motor	Health	Others	2011-12	2010-11	Fire	Marine	Motor	Health	Others	2011-12	2010-11
BAJAJ ALLIANZ	13021	6128	170298	35626	22396	247468	214965	6265	3223	147970	23697	9639	190795	170127	48.12	52.6	86.89	66.52	43.04	77.1	79.14
BHARTI AXA	521	430	45030	9345	1136	56463	31570	443	244	39034	7517	270	47507	27596	85.1	56.64	86.68	80.44	23.74	84.14	87.41
CHOLAMANDALAM	2893	1418	59031	17297	6274	86913	62737	1573	1102	48192	13234	1716	65818	48578	54.37	77.72	81.64	76.51	27.36	75.73	77.43
FUTURE GENERALI	1355	1108	35779	10554	3337	52133	32912	1573	839	28020	9032	1508	40973	27902	116.05	75.75	78.32	85.58	45.21	78.59	84.78
HDFC ERGO	2708	1502	53592	19621	14025	91447	60636	1620	2458	53111	13250	6203	76643	50988	59.83	163.65	99.1	67.53	44.23	83.81	84.09
ICICI LOMBARD	11459	5389	190185	109915	37952	354900	285616	9049	5157	224565	94739	26580	360091	273064	78.97	95.69	118.08	86.19	70.04	101.46	95.61
IFFCO TOKIO	5131	4010	98012	12613	13501	133268	113510	3859	3815	97682	10821	7189	123367	99046	75.21	95.15	99.66	85.79	53.24	92.57	87.26
L&T GENERAL	143	172	3687	402	485	4889	28	134	240	4091	737	534	5736	245	93.23	139.56	110.96	183.4	110.13	117.32	868.64
RAHEJA QBE	49	6	113	0	625	794	-175	32	12	173	0	200	417	183	65.37	195.25	152.55	0	31.99	52.53	-104.47
RELIANCE	3023	987	88021	19437	4841	116309	129380	2643	1029	101579	16672	4664	126587	133138	87.43	104.3	115.4	85.77	96.35	108.84	102.9
ROYAL SUNDARAM	1188	1244	84545	18515	5012	110503	87619	563	279	74259	9417	2042	86559	66022	47.39	22.39	87.83	50.86	40.73	78.33	75.35
SBI GENERAL	680	-19	2173	243	384	3461	-253	1230	24	3171	298	268	4993	564	181.05	-126.6	145.93	122.82	69.85	144.26	-222.74
SHRIRAM	241	21	53702	0	322	54286	33003	163	35	37486	0	152	37836	25508	67.82	171.08	69.8		47.2	69.7	77.29
TATA AIG	1858	13838	63851	9839	19045	108432	72669	1109	11219	64365	4885	4805	86383	54311	59.68	81.08	100.81	49.65	25.23	79.67	74.74
UNIVERSAL SOMPO	2914	197	15359	2554	3629	24654	19275	1384	222	16191	2620	1459	21876	14216	47.5	112.36	105.42	102.59	40.2	88.73	73.75
TOTAL	47183	36432	963378	265960	132965	1445919	1143493	31641	29899	939890	206920	67229	1275579	991490	67.06	82.07	97.56	77.8	50.56	88.22	86.71

Source: IRDAI annual reports.

Annexure 4

Case Study of BASIX in Community Health Insurance

BASIX represents a group of five entities which are:

Bhartiya Samruddhi Investments and Consulting Services, Ltd, a holding company;

Bhartiya Samruddhi Finance Limited (Samruddhi), a non-banking finance company;

Indian Grameen Services (IGS), a section 25 non-profit company;

Krishna Bhima Samruddhi Local Area Bank Limited (KBSLAB), a local area bank; and

Sarvodaya Nano Finance Ltd (Sarvodaya), registered by the Reserve Bank of India, a non-banking finance company, owned by women's self-help groups, and managed by BASICS Ltd.

BASIX began working in the life insurance sector in 2002. In May 2005, BASIX collaborated with Royal Sundaram Alliance (RSA) to expand into the health insurance business, offering risk coverage for total and permanent disability, critical illness and hospitalisation.

In March 2006, BASIX also launched a health product specifically for self-help group (SHG) members within the BASIX network. Operating within a partner-agent model, BASIX now has five insurance products: life, livestock, health, micro-enterprise and rainfall.

Health Insurance Products

BASIX offers two health products, both of which are reimbursement policies:

> These are Grameen Arogya Raksha and Self-Help Group Parivaar Beema. Both products are linked to credit and savings activities and are compulsory for the borrower but voluntary for the borrower's spouse. Grameen Arogya Raksha provides coverage for three categories of risks: critical illness, total and permanent disability due to accident and hospital cash to cover expenses related to hospitalisation. It is sold by the micro-credit lender, Bhartiya Samruddhi Finance Ltd (BSFL, or Samruddhi), one of the subsidiary companies of BASIX.

Originally the annual premium amount was Rs 136 for the borrower alone without an option to cover to the spouse. After one year of implementation the favourable experience suggested a reduction of the premium to half but instead a decision was made to cover both the borrower and the spouse for the same premium amount. Currently, the premium for the health insurance policy remains at Rs 68 per person or 136 for a couple. There is no coverage for other family members.

People are covered for as long as they are borrowing from BASIX and are not delinquent on their loan repayments.

There is no waiting period, no deductible and no co-payment at the time of hospitalisation.

The benefits offered through the insurance scheme are: hospitalisation cash benefit of Rs 300 per day up to 5 days, critical illness benefit of Rs 10,000, and Rs 25,000 total and permanent disability due to accident. There has been an expression of interest from insured clients for higher hospitalisation benefits, for outpatient benefits and for surgery benefits up to Rs 15,000. Features of the Current BASIX Health Insurance Program are given in Table 5.A4.1.

Table 5.A4.1 BASIX: Some Characteristics

Characteristic	Description
Owner and manager of scheme	BASIX, a for profit NGO
Administrator and TPA	BASIX manages claims processing but outsource to BPO
Distribution and marketing	Consumers are educated through BASIX staff
Service provider	Beneficiaries can use health services at any public or private facility
Starting date	2005 for health and 2002 for life insurance
Insurance term	Duration of loan payment. Not extended insurance if client is delinquent
Scope of operation	Eleven states
Participation	All using BASIX's loan services at a nominal premium

Source: https://basixindia.com/

Table 5.A4.1a BASIX: Some Additional Characteristics

Characteristic	Description
Insured unit	Coverage for borrower and spouse
Risk pooling	Risk is borne by the insurance company Royal Sundaram Alliance
Target market	Productive BPL borrowers of BASIX
Eligibility requirement	Qualification for getting loan from BASIX, limited to age 18–54
Annual premium rate	Rs. 68 per person per month (136 couples)
Premium collection	Monthly when loan repayment is made at specified community locations Grameen Arogya Rakesh critical illness Rs. 10,000 permanent total disability Rs. 25000 hospital cash Rs 300 per day up to Rs. 1500 (5 days per annum)
Benefits	SHG Parivar Beema Life Rs. 20,000 PTD: Rs. 20.000 hospital cash Rs. 1500
Exclusions	none
Claim settlement	Done at BASIX; approximately 50-60 days for reimbursement to the insured
Waiting period	No waiting period
Co-payment and user fees	none
Availing benefits	No pre-authorisation necessary
Financing	Premium to the insurance company and BAIX charges Rs. 10 per person for scheme administration

Source: https://basixindia.com/

Likewise, an overview of the Grameen Arogya Raksha Component of BASIX is presented below.

Table 5.A4.2 Grameen Arogya Raksha Component of BASIX

Target clients	Rural credit customers of BASIX and their spouses
Insurer	Royal Sundaram
Group or individual	Group
Policy holder	BSFL
Minimum entry age	18 years last birthday
Maximum age	54 years last birthday; exit age is 65
Policy benefits and sum insured	Critical illness Rs. 10,000; PTD, Rs. 25000, hospital cash Rs. 300 per day up to Rs. 1500 (5 days per annum)
Exclusions and waiting time	30 days waiting period for claiming hospital cash
Premium rate	Rs. 68 per year per person. Premium is paid monthly
Frequency of premium payment to insurance company	From disbursement date to last date of the month in which loan is closed
Coverage period	Coverage stops when loan repayment is overdue by 180 days from the last payment schedule date
Medical check-up	Not required

Source: https://basixindia.com/

Overview of the Self-Health Group Parivaar Beema of BASIX are also given as follows:

Table 5.A4.3 Self-Health Group Parivaar Beema of BASIX

Target clients	SHG which are institutional clients of BASIX
Insurer	AVIVA for life and Royal Sundaram for health
Group or individual	Group
Policy holder	Indian Grameen Services
Minimum entry age	18 years last birthday
Maximum age	54 years last birthday; exit age is 65
Policy benefits and sum insured	Life Rs. 20000 and PTD: Rs. 20000; Hospital cash Rs. 1500
Exclusions and waiting time	30 days waiting period for claiming hospital cash; first year suicide exclusion; no claim for life in first three months except in case of accidental death
Premium rate	Rs. 372 per year per member or Rs. 31 per month per person (this rate contains the premium for SHG group and spouse)
Frequency of premium payment to insurance company	Monthly or yearly option is available depending on the MIS system available within the local institution
Coverage period	12 months from the date of application
Medical check-up	Not required

Source: https://basixindia.com/

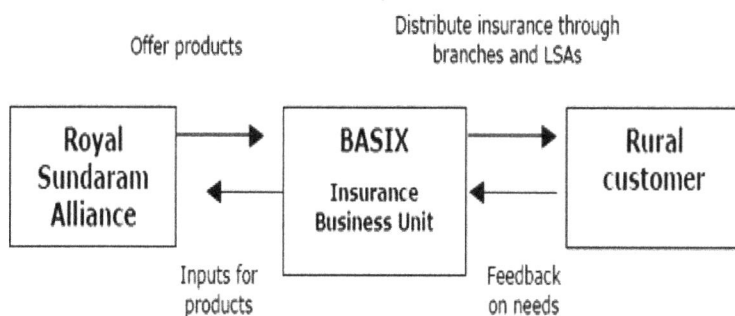

Figure 5.A4.1 Organisational Structure of BASIX Health Insurance.

Source: https://basixindia.com/

Table 5.A4.4 Number of BASIX Health Insurance Clients by Gender as of November 30, 2006

Age bracket	Female borrowers	Male spouses	Male borrowers	Female spouses	Total M and F
18–25	13,119	5311	15,842	10,124	44,396
25–35	32,475	26,631	40,678	23,984	13,768
35–45	29,679	22,746	30,453	20,093	102,971
45–54	10,658	10,744	13,868	5087	40,357
Total	85,931	65,432	100841	59,288	311,492

Source: https://basixindia.com/

Table 5.A4.5 Performance in Claims Servicing as of December 26, 2006

Insurance products	claims reported	claims settled	% of claims settled	claims in process	% of claims in process	claims rejected	% of claims rejected	claims amount paid (Rs. In million)
Life	1073	1010	94	56	5	7	1	14.6
Health	2399	1951	81	138	6	310	13	2.62
Livestock	899	802	89	39	4	58	6	6.18
Micro-enterprise shield	–	–	100	0	0	0	0	0.02
Total	4372	3764	86	233	375	375	9	23.42

Source: https://basixindia.com/

Karuna Trust Community Health Insurance

Karuna Trust was established in 1986 by Dr H. Sudarshan as a public charitable trust.

It is focused on a holistic, integrated, needs-based, participatory and bottom-up approach to development. The NGO works primarily with tribal, rural, and urban poor (both Scheduled Caste/Scheduled Tribes (SC/ST) and non-SC/ST BPL) taking into account cultural and regional differences and with emphasis on building skills, self-reliance and empowerment that enables communities to solve their own health problems.

The main focus areas are its numerous health projects and programmes, community development (including SHG development, microfinance, organic farming and vocational training), education and advocacy.

Karuna Trust was founded specifically to respond to the high prevalence of leprosy in Yelandur taluk of the Chamarajanagar district in Karnataka in 1986. After successful completion of the initial but limited leprosy eradication programme, the state government put Karuna Trust in charge of running its entire leprosy program for Yelandur taluk. This was followed by several other partnerships in which the NGO was charged with state responsibilities in exchange for a portion of the government budgets allocated to these areas.

Community Health Insurance Pilot

The community health insurance scheme (CHI), one of two pilot projects of UNDP and the Indian Ministry of Health, was conceived in 2001 as an experiment in community health financing. One pilot scheme was set up in West Bengal. The second pilot, selected because of a desire to work only with well-established and successful NGOs, resulted in partnering with Karuna Trust and the Center for Population Dynamics (CPD), a Bangalore-based research institution.

The Karuna Trust CHI experiment was unique and innovative in several ways:

- It augmented and built on the existing government infrastructure and to some degree compensated for its deficiencies;
- Benefits did not include the cost of provider services since these were supposed to be free at government facilities – instead, a daily cash benefit was paid during inpatient stays which was meant to lighten the burden of lost livelihood income while hospitalised; as such the benefit improved financial access and encouraged the insured to seek earlier, more timely treatment;
- A drug fund was set up at each accredited facility and was used to purchase required drugs needed over and above the basic drugs regularly stocked at each facility.

A benefit of Rs 50 per inpatient day was allocated towards purchasing drugs needed for the patient's treatment and not normally stocked in the PHC;

The Karuna Trust CHI experiment was unique and innovative in several ways:

Drug costs were lowered when Karuna Trust acquired quality generic drugs from reliable suppliers and supplied these in bulk to providers;

- The SHGs that Karuna Trust had helped to establish were each provided with a seed fund to be used for providing emergency loans to outpatients;
- Karuna Trust managed some of the public PHCs directly, thus ensuring quality care at these facilities; and
- As part of a wider preventive health programme that complemented the scheme, herbal gardens and Ayurvedic practices were promoted to preserve traditional and well-accepted treatments for minor ailments and prevention

The objectives of the CHI pilot included the following:

- Improve awareness and access to services through prepaid insurance;
- Enhance awareness and utilisation of government medical facilities;
- Motivate primary and secondary health care in a timely fashion;
- Develop and demonstrate working models of CHI for possible replication;
- Develop partnership experiences with the organised insurance sector; and
- Develop CHI through local government structures, SHGs and cooperative societies.

The objectives of the CHI pilot included the following:

- Improve awareness and access to services through prepaid insurance;
- Enhance awareness and utilisation of government medical facilities;
- Motivate primary and secondary health care in a timely fashion;
- Develop and demonstrate working models of CHI for possible replication;
- Develop partnership experiences with the organised insurance sector; and
- Develop CHI through local government structures, SHGs and cooperative societies.

The pilot scheme was initially limited to T. Narsipur taluk in Mysore district and Bailhongal taluk in Belgaum district. The target populations within these pilot areas were BPL SC/ST and non-SC/ST; more specifically these groups included landless labourers, rural self-employed, small and marginal farmers, unorganised agricultural seasonal labourers, construction labourers and forest dwelling tribes.

Karuna Trust made considerable inroads in the health sector in the [CHI project] area.

Scope and Phases of the Pilot CHI Project

Table 5.A4.6 Coverage and Experience in Phases I and II

Area	BPL SC/ ST	Non-SC/ ST	No. of participants	No. of claims	Total bed ays	Paid claims	Premium (rate@30)	Paid claims ratio
T. Narsipura taluk	82,546	2546	85,092	655	5490	54,900	2552,760	22
Bailhongal taluk	32,428	20,322	52,750	1719	12,241	1,224,100	1,582,500	77
Chamrajnagar district	33,716	–	33,716	402	3187	318,700	101,480	32
Belgaum taluk	59,496	–	59,496	339	1245	124,500	1,784,880	7
Total	208,186	2546	231,054	3115	22,163	2,216,300	6,931,620	32

Source: https://www.karuna.org

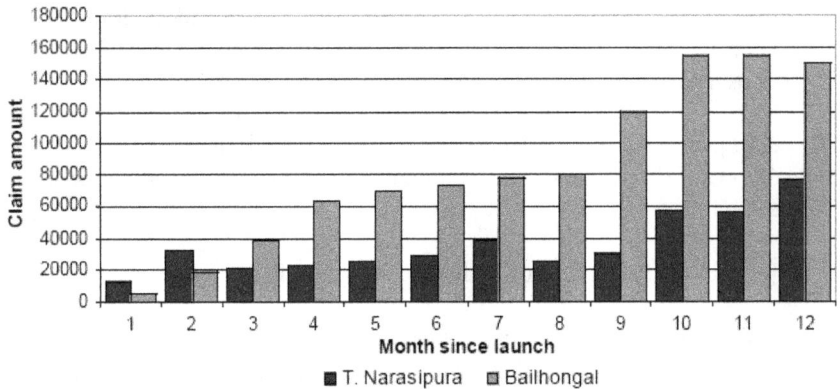

Figure 5.A4.2 Coverage and Experience in Different Phases of Karuna Trust Trends in Monthly Claims in Two Pilot Areas

Notes

1 Family floater health policies are umbrella health cover tailored for the entire family. A single premium is paid to obtain a cumulative health cover for the entire family and the amount of health coverage can be utilized for hospitalization expenses for a member of family.

2 The senior citizen policies are similar to individual health policies but come with stringent medical check-ups, high premiums, the higher waiting period for pre-existing illnesses and a greater number of exclusion clauses. These policies are usually bought by people who have already crossed 60 years of age but did not have any health insurance until then.

3 Top-up and super top-up policies are health policies which come with a "deductible" clause. These policies come into effect after the amount specified as the deductible is incurred as hospitalization expenses.

4 These policies are designed for people who are already diagnosed with certain diseases or are at high risk of getting certain diseases. The biggest advantage is that these policies cover illnesses like heart disease or cancer, which are usually avoided by many insurers. The premiums for such policies are high as the risk is high for the insurer.

5 The incurred claim ratios for both public and private sector individual companies is presented in Annexure 3, Tables 5.A3.3 and 5.A3.4.

6 International Labour Office (Universitas Programme). Extending social protection in health through community based health organizations: Evidence and challenges. Geneva: ILO, 2002.

7 World Health Organization. Macroeconomics and health: Investing in health for economic development. Geneva: World Health Organization,2002.

8 See, for instance, Ranson M. Kent, Community-based health insurance schemes in India: A review: Volume 16 Number 2 March/April 2003, pp. 1–17.

9 The Insurance Regulatory and Development Authority, annual report, 2011–12.

References

Dhingra, Reeta (2001), "NGOs and Health Insurance Schemes In India." *Health and Population- Perspectives and Issues* 24(4): 206–217.

Panda, Pradeep, Chakraborty, Arpita, Dror, David M, Bedi, Arjun S (2014) "Enrolment in community-based health insurance schemes in rural Bihar and Uttar Pradesh, India." *Health Policy and Planning* 29(8): 960–974

Ranson, M. Kent (2003). "Community-based health insurance schemes in India: A review." *The National Medical Journal of India* 16(2): 79–89.

Chapter 6

Demand for Health Insurance in India

Generally, it is presumed that health insurance will help to overcome excessive out of pocket expenses, which are sometimes a catastrophic proportion, and can lead to significant debt for a low income individual or household. As long back as 1963, the issue that patients may demand more health care if they are insured or the issue of a moral hazard were discussed (Arrow, 1963, 1968). Thus, presumably, high ethical responsibility on both the supply and the demand sides of medical care should prevail to avoid such a moral hazard effect of insurance. Thus, optimal health insurance should be actuarially fair to satisfy a risk averse individual to opt for a suitable insurance plan.[1] The supply and demand side of health insurance should also be such that optimal insurance plans are offered to satisfy risk averse individuals without the problems of either moral hazard or supplier induced demand. The latter is built with different reimbursement systems innate with various insurance plans like fee for service or others which allow cream skimming of insured patients.[2] In the Indian context, literature on demand for health care and health care insurance is scarce.[3]

In order to understand the dynamics of health insurance in India we used NFHS 4 data. The National Family Health Survey 2015–2016 (NFHS-4),[4] the fourth in the NFHS series, provides information on population, health and nutrition for India and in each State/Union territory. NFHS-4 fieldwork for India was conducted from January 20, 2015 to December 4, 2016 by 14 field agencies that gathered information from 601,509 households, 699,686 women and 112,122 men.

According to NFHS 4, at all-India level, the following situation prevails in regard to health insurance:

> In the case of urban areas, the health insurance coverage is slightly less at 28.2 percent, whereas it is slightly higher at 28.9 percent in rural areas (Tables 6.1).

To understand the socio-economic correlations of health insurance we conducted logit analysis and also derived marginal effects, or average elasticities,

DOI: 10.4324/9781032615660-6

Table 6.1 Overall Health Insurance Coverage in India (2015–2016)

Member of Household Covered by a Health Scheme or Health Insurance		
All India	*Rural*	*Urban*
28.7	28.9	28.2

Source: NFHS 4.

in regard to different independent variables used in analysing the results. The logit analysis is used here due to the fact that we are interested in looking into health insurance choices as a dependent variable. An individual or household may decide to go for a particular health insurance plan being offered by the public or private sector based upon his/her circumstances, which are largely related to socio-economic factors. Since the choice is between two types, either to opt or not to opt for a particular health insurance plan or a binary choice variable as a dependent one, this analysis involving logit regressions is considered useful. Thus, we use the choice of a particular health insurance plan as the dependent variable and analyse using basic socio-economic variables, including income or wealth index from NFHS 4 survey, sex of individual, age and education levels of individuals. We also take into account rural or urban location of individuals by segregating the rural and urban population covered in NFHS survey. It is worth mentioning that the survey gives numeric value one to five for wealth index which is denoted as poorest, poorer, middle, richer and richest, respectively. Thus, to consider BPL, we included respondents with wealth index value as one. From the numeric value of wealth index the respondents falling into two to five wealth index values were denoted by us as above BPL population. Likewise, we segregated the respondents according to NFHS criteria into educated or uneducated based upon the respondents' numeric value belonging to middle, secondary or higher education (educated) and others (uneducated) respectively. Thus, four sets of results are provided below which are termed as below BPL and uneducated respondents rural, or urban and above BPL and educated respondents belonging to rural and urban areas separately. We presume the results of our analysis may provide us with an idea of what are the main socio-economic correlations of making a choice about opting for an insurance plan. Thus, we look into different types of health insurance plans that the NFHS 4 survey covers which, among others, include, ESIS, CGHS, State Health Insurance Plan (SHI), RSBY, Community Health Insurance (CHI) and Privately Purchased Health Insurance Plan (PHI). Out of these plans, ESIS and CGHS require certain basic requirements and there is no choice for others not belonging to the above two categories, which are predefined by their occupation either in central government, or in factory sector with certain income slabs. Therefore, we only focus on the other four types of health insurance decisions involving either SHI, RSBY, CHI or PHI. The results of our logit analysis are discussed below.

Results for Poorest (BPL) and Uneducated Rural Households

Table 6.2 provides the results of a choice between no health insurance or any health insurance. We can observe that signs of Rural Wealth Index (RWI), Highest Education Level attained by the individuals (HEL) and age are positive and significant also. This indicates that one may decide to go for a health insurance based on these factors. The coefficients are, however, low (second column Table 6.2). From these coefficients, marginal effects or elasticities with respect to these explanatory variables (at the average values) are presented in Table 6.2(a). Though the marginal effects are statistically significant, magnitude is very low. This confirms that health insurance demand is one belonging to the set of essential goods or services.

Table 6.2 Any Health Insurance

Logistic regression

Number of obs = 96,525;			LR chi2(3) = 322.44
Prob> chi2 = 0.000;			
Log likelihood = -51866.134			Pseudo R2 = 0.0031

HI	Coef.	z	P>|z|
RWI	0.127	7.46	0.000
HEL	0.079	8.18	0.000
AGE	0.008	14.69	0.000
Constant	-1.77	-51.26	0.000

Source: Estimated.

Table 6.2(a) Any Health Insurance (Marginal Effects)

Conditional marginal effects for HI in Table 1
Number of obs =96,525
Model VCE: OIM
Delta-method

	ey/ex	z	P>z
RWI	0.124	7.46	0.000
HEL	0.019	8.18	0.000
AGE	0.286	14.67	0.000

Source: Estimated.

The results of logit for RSBY (Table 6.3 and 6.3(a)) for the rural BPL and uneducated respondents also suggest significant coefficients for RWI and age with a negative sign. It implies that sometimes poor living conditions and age may impede enrolment in the scheme. The elasticity is also low here, indicating restricted nature of choice (Table 6.3 and 6.3(a)). A similar restrictive situation is depicted for State Health Insurance (Table 6.4 and 6.4(a)).

Further, a look at the results of health insurance choice pertaining to employer provided insurance also indicates a negative effect of age factor and a high elasticity value (1.91, Table 6.56.5(a)). This suggests that one may opt for another health insurance plan based on maturity of respondent.

The negative impact of age factor is also noticeable for choices in regard to private health insurance (Table 6.6) and low marginal impacts of explanatory variables (Table 6.6(a)).

However, the results for female respondents in BPL sample indicates a high and positive significant coefficient and elasticity with respect to RWI (Tables 6.7 and 6.7(a)). This may suggest that income has a significant positive impact on the decision to opt for private health insurance, particularly in females. This kind of impact is absent, however, for females in regard to health insurance provision by the employer (Table 6.8 and 6.8(a)).

Table 6.3 RSBY

Logistic regression   Number of obs =21,775
LR chi2(3) =80.60
Prob> chi2 =0.0000
Log likelihood = -14270.314   Pseudo R2 =0.0028

RSBY	Coef.	z	P>z
RWI	-0.222	-7.21	0
HEL	0.01	0.51	0.611
AGE	-0.005	-5.08	0
_cons	1.094	16.29	0

Source: Estimated.

Table 6.3(a) RSBY (Marginal Effects)

Conditional marginal effects for Table 2
Number of obs = 21,775
Model VCE: OIM
Delta-method

	ey/ex	z	P>z
RWI	-0.1048	-7.21	0
HEL	0.0013	0.51	0.61
AGE	-0.096	-5.08	0

Source: Estimated.

Table 6.4 State HIS

Logistic regression   Number of obs =21,775
LR chi2(3) =62.11
Prob> chi2 =0.0000
Log likelihood = -14291.524   Pseudo R2 =0.0022

State HI	Coef.	z	P>z
RWI	0.161	5.24	0.000
HEL	0.021	1.07	0.283
AGE	0.005	5.71	0.000
Constant	-1.054	-15.71	0.000

Source: Estimated.

Table 6.4(a) State HIS (Marginal effects)

Conditional marginal effects
for Table 3
Number of obs =21,775
Model VCE: OIM
Delta-method

	ey/ex	z	P>z
RWI	0.131	5.23	0.000
HEL	0.004	1.07	0.283
AGE	0.186	5.7	0.000

Source: Estimated.

Table 6.5 HITEMPloyer

Logistic regression   Number of obs =21,775
LR chi2(3) =11.78
Prob> chi2 =0.0082
Log likelihood = -234.81   Pseudo R2 =0.0245

HITEMP	Coef.	z	P>z
RWI	0.728	2.030	0.042
HEL	-0.512	-1.250	0.211
AGE	-0.038	-2.680	0.007
_cons	-5.569	-6.770	0.000

Source: Estimated.

Table 6.5(a) HITEMPloyer (Marginal Effects)

Delta-method
Conditional marginal effects   Number of obs =21,775
Model VCE: OIM

	ey/ex	Z	P(z)
RWI	0.93576	2.03	0.042
HEL	-0.173	-1.25	0.212
AGE	-1.9113	-2.68	0.007

Source: Estimated.

Table 6.6 Private Health Insurance

Logistic regression   Number of obs = 21,775
LR chi2(3) = 2.59
Prob> chi2 = 0.4599
Log likelihood = -447.33168   Pseudo R2 = 0.0029

PrHI	Coef.	Z	P>z
RWI	0.277	1.070	0.285
HEL	0.156	1.290	0.198
AGE	-0.003	-0.290	0.770
_cons	-6.090	-10.510	0.000

Source: Estimated.

Table 6.6(a) Private Health Insurance (Marginal Effects)

Delta-method
Conditional marginal effects Private Health Insurance
Number of obs =21,775
Model VCE: OIM

	ey/ex	z	P>z
RWI	0.356	1.07	0.285
HEL	0.053	1.29	0.198
AGE	-0.133	-0.29	0.77

Source: Estimated.

Table 6.7 Private Health Insurance for Females

Logistic regression   Number of obs =4,149
LR chi2(3) =12.30
Prob> chi2 =0.0064
Log likelihood = -58.039   Pseudo R2 =0.0958

PriHIF	Coef.	z	P>z
RWI	1.407	1.950	0.052
HEL	0.687	4.240	0.000
AGE	0.028	1.170	0.241
_cons	-9.940	-5.260	0.000

Source: Estimated.

Table 6.7(a) Private Health Insurance for Females
(Marginal Effects)

Delta-method
Conditional marginal effects   Number of obs =4,149
Model VCE: OIM

PriHIF	ey/ex	z	P>z
RWI	1.802	1.950	0.052
HEL	0.086	4.230	0.000
AGE	1.488	1.170	0.241

Source: Estimated.

Table 6.8 HITEMPloyer for Females

Logistic regression   Number of obs =4,149
LR chi2(3) =0.14
Prob> chi2 =0.9873
Log likelihood = -51.619   Pseudo R2 =0.0013

HITEMP	Coef.	z	P>z
RWI	0.017	0.020	0.984
HEL	0.113	0.160	0.874
AGE	0.009	0.350	0.725
_cons	-6.922	-3.710	0.000

Source: Estimated.

Table 6.8(a) HITEMPloyer for Females (Marginal Effects)

Delta-method
Conditional marginal effects   Number of obs =4,149
Model VCE: OIM

	ey/ex	z	P>z
RWI	0.022	0.020	0.984
HEL	0.014	0.160	0.874
AGE	0.493	0.350	0.725

Source: Estimated.

Results for above BPL Rural Households

Results for above BPL (ABPL) individuals in rural areas are presented in Tables 6.9 to 6.14. The coefficients of income or RWI varies from .076 (for HI) to -.396 (for RSBY). The signs and significance also change across schemes for variables of sex, education and age. Both the impact and marginal impact in any of the schemes including HI, SHI, CHI, RSBY is very low (Tables 6.9 to 6.12 and Tables 6.9(a) to 6.12(a)). Only a difference of high impact of income variables is noticeable for private health insurance across the respondents in aggregate and for female respondents also (Tables 6.13-6.14 and 6.13(a)–6.14(a)). The magnitude of coefficient of income as well as elasticities is higher than three (Tables 6.13(a) ad 6.14(a)). This indicates that income affects private insurance purchase decisions, however for other types it really does not matter that much.

Results for Poorest (BPL) Urban Households

The results of BPL individuals are presented in Tables 6.15 to 6.21. In these results, only education and age have appeared significant with low

Table 6.9 HI ABPL

Logistic regression   Number of obs =216,881
LR chi2(4) =643.75
Prob> chi2 =0.0000
Log likelihood = -128105.52   Pseudo R2 =0.0025

HI	Coef.	z	P>
RWI	0.076	15.910	0.000
HEL	-0.117	-16.620	0.000
SEX	0.089	5.050	0.000
Age	0.002	6.720	0.000
cons	1.232528 .	37.740	0.000

Source: Estimated.

Table 6.9(a) HI ABPL (Elasticities)

Delta-method
Conditional marginal effects   Number of obs =216,881
Model VCE: OIM

	ey/ex	z	P>z
RWI	0.208	15.900	0.000
HEL	-0.157	-16.600	0.000
SEX	0.069	5.050	0.000
Age	0.082	6.720	0.000

Source: Estimated.

Table 6.10 SHI

Logistic regression   Number of obs =59,153
LR chi2(4) =761.17
Prob> chi2 =0.0000
Log likelihood = -40155.432   Pseudo R2 =0.0094

SHI	Coef.	z	P>
RWI	0.079	9.280	0.000
HEL	-0.086	-7.140	0.000
SEX	-0.262	-8.540	0.000
Age	-0.017	-25.820	0.000
_cons	0.705	12.160	0.000

Source: Estimated.

Table 6.10(a) SHI (Elasticities)

Delta-method
Conditional marginal effects   Number of obs =59,153
Model VCE: OIM

	ey/ex	Z	P>z
RWI	0.171	9.270	0.000
HEL	-0.088	-7.140	0.000
SEX	-0.160	-8.530	0.000
Age	-0.464	-25.630	0.000

Source: Estimated.

Table 6.11 RSBY

Logistic regression   Number of obs =59,153
LR chi2(4) =2709.91
Prob> chi2 =0.0000
Log likelihood = -39138.551   Pseudo R2 =0.0335

RSBY	Coef.	z	P>z
RWI	-0.396	-45.310	0.000
HEL	-0.097	-8.060	0.000
SEX	0.185	6.050	0.000
Age	0.013	19.140	0.000
_cons	0.603	10.400	0.000

Source: Estimated.

Table 6.11(a) RSBY(Elasticities)

Delta-method
Conditional marginal effects   Number of obs=59,153
Model VCE: OIM

	ey/ex	z	P>z
RWI	0.860	-44.430	0.000
HEL	-0.100	-8.050	0.000
SEX	0.114	6.050	0.000
Age	0.348	19.070	0.000

Source: Estimated.

Table 6.12 CHI

Logistic regression   Number of obs =59,153
LR chi2(4) =28.11
Prob> chi2 =0.0000
Log likelihood = -2068.6922   Pseudo R2 =0.0067

CHI	Coef.	Z	P>z
RWI	0.211	3.640	0.000
HEL	0.098	1.480	0.138
SEX	-0.229	-1.050	0.293
Age	0.011	2.520	0.012
_cons	-6.445	16.380	0.000

Source: Estimated.

Table 6.12(a) CHI Elasticities

Delta-method
Conditional marginal effects   Number of obs =59,153
Model VCE: OIM

	ey/ex	z	P>z
RWI	0.804	3.640	0.000
HEL	0.177	1.480	0.138
SEX	-0.246	-1.050	0.293
Age	0.503	2.520	0.012

Source: Estimated.

Table 6.13 Private Insurance

Logistic regression   Number of obs =59,153
LR chi2(4) =895.77
Prob> chi2 =0.0000
Log likelihood = -6675.8494   Pseudo R2 =0.0629

Private IN	Coef.	z	P>z
RWI	0.815	23.100	0.000
HEL	0.260	9.830	0.000
SEX	0.023	0.240	0.809
Age	0.006	2.920	0.004
_cons	-7.861	37.240	0.000

Source: Estimated.

Table 6.13(a) Private Insurance (Elasticities)

Delta-method
Conditional marginal effects   Number of obs =59,153
Model VCE: OIM

	ey/ex	Z	P>Z
RWI	3.061	22.880	0.000
HEL	0.462	9.820	0.000
SEX	0.024	0.240	0.809
Age	0.277	2.920	0.004

Source: Estimated.

Table 6.14 Private Insurance Females

Logistic regression   Number of obs =4,971
LR chi2(3) =83.27
Prob> chi2 =0.0000
Log likelihood = -567.56846   Pseudo R2 =0.0683

PriIF	Coef.	z	P>z
RWI	0.923	6.880	0.000
HEL	0.242	2.770	0.006
AGE	0.013	1.920	0.055
_cons	-8.616	-12.400	0.000

Source: Estimated.

Table 6.14(a) Private Insurance Females (Elasticities)

Delta-method
Conditional marginal effects   Number of obs =4,971
Model VCE: OIM

PriIF	ey/ex	z	P>z
RWI	3.560	6.810	0.000
HEL	0.388	2.770	0.006
AGE	0.596	1.920	0.055

Source: Estimated.

coefficients for HI, SHI, RSBY, CHI and employer provided health insurance schemes. Likewise, the results for marginal impact also indicate low elasticities (Tables 6.15(a) to 6.21(a)). There are probably very limited choices for BPL urban respondents, which is reflected in these results. Even the private health insurance has similarly low coefficients (Tables 6.20 and 6.20(a)), in contrast to their rural counterparts. There are slight differences of education variable with a higher value at 1.968 but an insignificant difference for females in the urban BPL population is noted (Table 6.21 and 6.21(a)).

Results for above BPL Urban Households

The results of above BPL urban individuals are presented in Tables 6.21–6.25 . More often a uniformity of statistically significant coefficient of income (or Urban Wealth Index) is noticeable for all types of health insurance plans. The coefficient for this variable varies from .080 (for HI, Table 6.21) to 0.191(for CHI, Table 6.24) to .653(for Phi, Table 6.25). For two schemes, namely SHI and RSBY, the impact coefficient of income is negative also

Table 6.15 Any Health Insurance (Urban BPL)

Logistic regression   Number of obs =5,383
LR chi2(3) =31.42
Prob> chi2 =0.0000
Log likelihood = -2733.0212   Pseudo R2 =0.0057

HI	Coef.	z	P>
HEL	0.116	3.220	0.001
SEX	0.066	0.840	0.401
AGE	0.011	4.650	0.000
_cons	-1.984	-14.170	0.000

Source: Estimated.

Table 6.15(a) Any Health Insurance (Urban BPL)
            (Elasticities)

Delta-method
Conditional marginal effects   Number of obs =5,383
Model VCE : OIM

HI	ey/ex	Z	P>Z
HEL	0.031	3.220	0.001
SEX	0.066	0.840	0.401
AGE	0.407	4.640	0.000

Source: Estimated.

Table 6.16 State Health Insurance (Urban BPL)

Logistic regression   Number of obs =1,102
LR chi2(3) =8.67
Prob> chi2 =0.0340
Log likelihood = -738.60254   Pseudo R2 =0.0058

SHI	Coef.	z	P>z
SEX	0.186	1.310	0.189
HEL	0.148	1.900	0.057
AGE	0.008	1.900	0.057
_cons	-1.118	-4.030	0.000

Source: Estimated.

Table 6.16(a) State Health Insurance (Urban BPL)

Delta-method
Conditional marginal effects   Number of obs =1,102
Model VCE: OIM

	ey/ex	Z	P>Z
SEX	0.142	1.310	0.190
HEL	0.033	1.900	0.058
AGE	0.256	1.900	0.058

Source: Estimated.

Table 6.17 RSBY (Urban BPL)

Logistic regression   Number of obs=1,102
LR chi2(3) =13.63
Prob> chi2 =0.0035
Log likelihood = -748.61833   Pseudo R2 =0.0090

RSBY	Coef.	z	P>Z
HEL	-0.180	-2.210	0.027
AGE	-0.011	-2.460	0.014
SEX	-0.233	-1.660	0.098
_cons	1.166	4.220	0.000

Source: Estimated.

Table 6.17(a) RSBY (Urban BPL) (elasticities)

Delta-method
Conditional marginal effects   Number of obs = 1,102
Model VCE : OIM

	ey/ex	z	P>z
HEL	0.030	-2.200	0.028
AGE	0.241	-2.460	0.014
SEX	0.130	-1.650	0.098

Source: Estimated.

Table 6.18 HITEMP(Urban BPL)

Logistic regression   Number of obs =1,102
LR chi2(2) =1.08
Prob> chi2 =0.5841
Log likelihood = -14.083976   Pseudo R2 =0.0368

HITEMPL	Coef.	z	P>z
HEL	0.200	0.370	0.708
AGE	0.052	1.000	0.319
_cons	-9.257	-2.840	0.004

Source: Estimated.

Table 6.18(a) HITEMP(Urban BPL) (Elasticities)

Delta-method
Conditional marginal effects   Number of obs =1,102
Model VCE : OIM

ey/ex	. Err.	Z	P>Z
HEL	0.076	0.370	0.708
AGE	2.597	1.000	0.319

Source: Estimated.

Table 6.19 PrHI(Urban BPL)

Logistic regression   Number of obs =1,102
LR chi2(3) =1.62
Prob> chi2 =0.6539
Log likelihood = -25.655022   Pseudo R2 =0.0307

PrHI	Coef.	Z	P>z
HEL	0.325	1.120	0.261
AGE	-0.004	-0.100	0.919
SEX	1.179	1.080	0.279
_cons	-7.232	-3.130	0.002

Source: Estimated.

Table 6.19(a) PrHI(Urban BPL) (Elasticities)

Delta-method
Conditional marginal effects   Number of obs =1,102
Model VCE: OIM

	ey/ex	Z	P>Z
HEL	0.122	1.120	0.262
AGE	-0.188	-0.100	0.919
SEX	1.506	1.080	0.279

Source: Estimated.

Table 6.20 PrHI(Urban BPL) (Females)

Logistic regression   Number of obs =310
LR chi2(2) =2.21
Prob> chi2 =0.3319
Log likelihood = -10.97733   Pseudo R2 =0.0913

PrHI	Coef.	z	P>z
HEL	1.968	1.360	0.173
AGE	-0.031	-0.580	0.559
_cons	-3.988	-1.420	0.157

Source: Estimated.

Table 6.20(a) PrHI (Urban BPL) (Females) (Elasticities)

Delta-method
Conditional marginal effects   Number of obs =310
Model VCE: OIM

	ey/ex	Z	P>Z
HEL	0.221	1.360	0.174
AGE	-1.692	-0.580	0.559

Source: Estimated.

(Tables 6.22 and 6.23). However, positive and high elasticity is noted for private health insurance choice for urban aggregate above PL respondents, as well as females in the same group of urban respondents (Tables 6.25a and 6.26a).

Thus, these results generally indicate that individuals have more choice for private health insurance commensurate with their higher income levels. For other types of insurance schemes from the public sector, the individual does

Table 6.21 Any Health Insurance (Urban Above BPL)

Logistic regression   Number of obs =140,546
LR chi2(4) =705.03
Prob> chi2 =0.0000
Log likelihood = -82249.995   Pseudo R2 =0.0043

HI	Coef.	z	P>Z
UWI	0.080	16.980	0.000
HEL	0.025	3.050	0.002
SEX	0.049	2.500	0.013
AGE	0.006	13.310	0.000
_cons	-1.626	-45.080	0.000

Source: Estimated.

Table 6.21(a) Any Health Insurance (Urban Above BPL) (Elasticities)

Delta-method
Conditional marginal effects   Number of obs =140,546
Model VCE: OIM

	ey/ex	Z	P>Z
HEL	0.038	3.050	0.002
SEX	0.039	2.500	0.013
AGE	0.213	13.300	0.000

Source: Estimated.

Table 6.22 State Health Insurance (Urban Above BPL)

Logistic regression   Number of obs =37,407
LR chi2(4) =1303.64
Prob> chi2 =0.0000
Log likelihood = -24471.218   Pseudo R2 =0.0259

HIState	Coef.	z	P>z
UWI	-0.213	-24.590	0.000
HEL	-0.112	-7.040	0.000
SEX	-0.103	-2.950	0.003
AGE	-0.011	-13.110	0.000
_cons	1.167	17.100	0.000

Source: Estimated.

Table 6.22(a) State Health Insurance (Urban Above
            BPL) (Elasticities)

Delta-method
Conditional marginal effects   Number of obs =37,407
Model VCE: OIM

	ey/ex	z	P>Z
UWI	0.422	-24.330	0.000
HEL	-0.143	-7.030	0.000
SEX	-0.069	-2.950	0.003
AGE	-0.338	-13.060	0.000

Source: Estimated.

Table 6.23 RSBY (Urban Above BPL)

Logistic regression   Number of obs =37,407
LR chi2(4) =3409.79
Prob> chi2 =0.0000
Log likelihood = -19289.905   Pseudo R2 =0.0812

RSBY	Coef.	z	P>z
UWI	-0.433	-41.520	0.000
HEL	-0.300	-14.900	0.000
SEX	0.306	8.110	0.000
AGE	0.012	12.410	0.000
_cons	-0.135	-1.730	-0.084

Source: Estimated.

Table 6.23(a) RSBY (Urban Above BPL) (Elasticities)

Delta-method
Conditional marginal effects   Number of obs =37,407
Model VCE: OIM

	ey/ex	Z	P>Z
UWI	-1.094	-40.040	0.000
HEL	-0.489	-14.810	0.000
SEX	0.263	8.110	0.000
AGE	0.470	12.380	0.000

Source: Estimated.

Table 6.24 CHI (Urban Above BPL)

Logistic regression   Number of obs =37,407
LR chi2(4) =24.91
Prob> chi2 =0.0001
Log likelihood = -1984.9656   Pseudo R2 =0.0062

CHI	Coef.	z	P>z
UWI	0.191	4.260	0.000
HEL	0.023	0.310	0.760
SEX	0.000	0.000	1.000
AGE	0.001	0.120	0.902
_cons	-5.388	5.630	0.000

Source: Estimated.

Table 6.24(a) CHI (Urban Above BPL) (Elasticities)

Delta-method
Conditional marginal effects   Number of obs =37,407
Model VCE: OIM

	ey/ex	z	P>z
UWI	0.618	4.260	0.000
HEL	0.048	0.310	0.760
SEX	0.000	0.000	1.000
AGE	0.026	0.120	0.902

Source: Estimated.

Table 6.25 PrHI (Urban Above BPL)

Logistic regression   Number of obs =37,407
LR chi2(4) =1986.45
Prob> chi2 =0.0000
Log likelihood = 9455.301   Pseudo R2 =0.0951

PrHI	Coef.	z	P>z
UWI	0.653	33.370	0.000
HEL	0.231	9.260	0.000
SEX	0.002	0.040	0.971
AGE	0.000	0.180	0.856
_cons	-5.442	9.340	0.000

Source: Estimated.

Table 6.25(a) PrHI (Urban Above BPL) (Elasticities)

Delta-method
Conditional marginal effects   Number of obs =37,407
Model VCE: OIM

	ey/ex	Z	P>Z
UWI	2.008	32.380	0.000
HEL	0.459	9.240	0.000
SEX	0.003	0.040	0.971
AGE	0.013	0.180	0.856

Source: Estimated.

Table 6.26 PrHI Females (Urban Above BPL)

Logistic regression   Number of obs =4,096
LR chi2(3) =170.87
Prob> chi2 =0.0000
Log likelihood = -922.89411   Pseudo R2 =0.0847

PrHIF	Coef. S	z	P>z
UWI	0.616	10.570	0.000
HEL	0.167	2.370	0.018
AGE	0.006	1.260	0.207
_cons	-5.466	-15.530	0.000

Source: Estimated.

Table 6.26(a) PrHI Females (Urban Above BPL)

Delta-method
Conditional marginal effects   Number of obs =4,096
Model VCE: OIM

	ey/ex	Z	P>z
UWI	1.798	10.310	0.000
HEL	0.288	2.370	0.018
AGE	0.299	1.260	0.207

Source: Estimated.

seem to exercise significant choice. Besides, education or sex variables also seem to have some impact on health insurance state sector schemes.

Further, in order to see if the nature of choice for individuals pertaining to health insurance schemes differs from aggregate all India rural or urban level to a state level analysis, we also attempted a similar analysis for a low-income state, using Madhya Pradesh as a case study. The results of the state level analysis from NFHS 4 data for Madhya Pradesh are presented in Tables 6.27 to 6.44(a)– and 6.276.44(a).

Results for MP

Results for MP Urban Poorest Uneducated

The results for MP pertaining to BPL uneducated respondents are presented in Tables 6.27 to 6.29 and 6.27(a)–6.29(a). These results relate to three schemes, namely SHI, RSBY and PHI. We notice that none of the three explanatory variables chosen in logit analysis namely sex, age and education

Table 6.27 SHI MP

Logistic regression   Number of obs =199
LR chi2(3) =3.58
Prob> chi2 =0.3102
Log likelihood = -122.43798   Pseudo R2 =0.0144

SHI	Coef.	z	P>z
SEX	0.364	0.920	0.358
AGE	-0.014	-1.230	0.218
EDU	0.224	1.150	0.250
const.	0.932	1.370	0.172

Source: Estimated.

Table 6.27(a) SHI MP

Delta-method
Average marginal effects   Number of obs =199
Model VCE: OIM

SHI	ey/ex	Z	P>Z
SEX	0.139	0.940	0.346
AGE	-0.228	-1.180	0.236
EDU	0.025	1.540	0.123

Source: Estimated.

for the state, relating to BPL urban respondents, is significant and there is variability in signs of these coefficients from SHI to PHI (Tables 6.27 to 6.29). Only in the results of PHI, age and education are both positive yet insignificant (Table 6.29). The elasticity (=11.577) is also high for PHI in regard to age (but statistically insignificant) (Table 6.29(a)).

Table 6.28 RSBY MP

Logistic regression   Number of obs =199
LR chi2(3) =4.68
Prob> chi2=0.1965
Log likelihood = -112.9942   Pseudo R2 =0.0203

RSBY	Coef.	z	P>z
SEX	-0.401	-0.960	0.337
AGE	0.018	1.500	0.133
EDU	-0.280	-1.180	0.240
Cons	-1.319	-1.810	0.710

Source: Estimated

Table 6.28(a) RSBY MP

Delta-method
Average marginal effects   Number of obs =199
Model VCE: OIM

RSBY	ey/ex	Z	P>Z
SEX	-0.361	-0.950	0.344
AGE	0.646	1.530	0.127
EDU	-0.114	-1.110	0.268

Source: Estimated.

Table 6.29 PHI MP

Logistic regression   Number of obs =199
LR chi2(2) =3.93
Prob> chi2 =0.1398
Log likelihood = -4.323508   Pseudo R2 =0.3127

PHI	Coef.	z	P>z
AGE	0.232	1.190	0.235
EDU	0.614	0.890	0.373
cons	-21.094	-1.400	0.160

Source: Estimated.

MP above BPL Urban Results

For above BPL urban respondents of MP, the results are presented in Tables 6.30–6.34 and 6.30(a)–6.34(a).

We notice that the income variable, or Urban Wealth Index (UWI), is negative and significant for SHI and RSBY (Tables 6.30-6.31). It is positive

Table 6.29(a) PHI

Delta-method
Average marginal effects   Number of obs =199
Model VCE: OIM

PHI	ey/ex	Z	P>Z
AGE	11.577	1.190	0.234
EDU	0.299	0.900	0.367

Source: Estimated.

Table 6.30 SHI MP ABPL Urban

Logistic regression   Number of obs =2,876
LR chi2(4) =463.92
Prob> chi2 =0.0000
Log likelihood = -1750.9977   Pseudo R2 =0.1170

SHI	Coef.	z	P>z
UWI	-0.550	-16.380	0.000
SEX	0.063	0.410	0.685
AGE	0.002	0.600	0.547
EDU	-0.266	-5.060	0.000
cons	2.296	8.650	0.000

Source: Estimated.

Table 6.30(a) SHI MP ABPL Urban

Delta-method
Average marginal effects   Number of obs =2,876
Model VCE: OIM

SHI	ey/ex	Z	P>Z
UWI	-0.931	-14.460	0.000
SEX	0.031	0.410	0.685
AGE	0.045	0.600	0.546
EDU	-0.272	-4.890	0.000

Source: Estimated.

but insignificant for CHI (Table 6.32). However, it is positive and significant for PHI (Table 6.33). Further private health insurance choice depicts high responsiveness in regard to income of these above BPL respondents of MP (Table 6.33(a)). This result of private health insurance in MP is in line

Table 6.31 RSBY MP ABPL Urban

Logistic regression   Number of obs =2,876
LR chi2(4) =92.91
Prob> chi2 =0.0000
Log likelihood = -791.21179   Pseudo R2 =0.0555

RSBY	Coef.	z	P>z
UWI	-0.492	-8.750	0.000
SEX	-0.108	-0.400	0.686
AGE	-0.006	-1.140	0.252
EDU	0.131	1.820	0.069
cons	-0.857	-2.030	0.042

Source: Estimated.

Table 6.31(a) RSBY MP ABPL Urban

Delta-method
Average marginal effects   Number of obs =2,876
Model VCE: OIM

RSBY	ey/ex	Z	P>Z
UWI	-1.440	-8.590	0.000
SEX	-0.106	-0.400	0.686
AGE	-0.284	-1.140	0.253
EDU	0.244	1.830	0.068

Source: Estimated.

Table 6.32 CHI MP ABPL Urban

Logistic regression   Number of obs =2,876
LR chi2(4) =7.50
Prob> chi2 =0.1116
Log likelihood = -232.11231   Pseudo R2 =0.0159

CHI	Coef.	z P	>z
UWI	0.180	1.530	0.125
SEX	0.689	1.550	0.122
AGE	0.003	0.210	0.836
EDU	0.189	1.330	0.182
cons	-6.003	-6.840	0.000

Source: Estimated.

with all-India urban results discussed above. However, the results of female respondents in MP in this group of above BPL respondents are different for private health insurance, which are not statistically significant and depict low responsiveness of PHI in regard to income (Tables 6.34 and 6.34(a)).

Table 6.32(a) CHI MP ABPL Urban

Delta-method
Average marginal effects   Number of obs =2,876
Model VCE: OIM

CHI	ey/ex	Z	P>Z
UWI	0.553	1.540	0.124
SEX	0.729	1.550	0.122
AGE	0.119	0.210	0.836
EDU	0.376	1.340	0.181

Source: Estimated.

Table 6.33 PHI MP ABPL Urban

Logistic regression   Number of obs =2,876
LR chi2(4) =100.81
Prob> chi2 =0.0000
Log likelihood = -592.52032   Pseudo R2 =0.0784

PHI	Coef.	z	P>z
UWI	0.560	7.570	0.000
SEX	-0.058	-0.180	0.860
AGE	0.002	0.380	0.707
EDU	0.227	2.700	0.007
cons	-5.361	-9.600	0.000

Source: Estimated.

Table 6.33(a) PHI MP ABPL Urban

Delta-method
Average marginal effects   Number of obs=2,876
Model VCE: OIM

PHI	ey/ex	Z	P>z
UWI	1.619	7.650	0.000
SEX	-0.059	-0.180	0.860
AGE	0.111	0.380	0.707
EDU	0.427	2.710	0.007

Source: Estimated.

Table 6.34 PHI ONLY FEMALES MP ABPL Urban

Logistic regression   Number of obs =218
LR chi2(3) =2.84
Prob> chi2 =0.4169
Log likelihood = -42.150038   Pseudo R2 =0.0326

PHI F	Coef.	z	P>z
UWI	0.317	1.270	0.204
AGE	-0.005	-0.190	0.851
EDU	0.165	0.690	0.490
cons	-4.041	-2.610	0.009

Source: Estimated.

Table 6.34(a) PHI ONLY FEMALES MP ABPL Urban

Delta-method
Average marginal effects   Number of obs=218
Model VCE: OIM

PHI F	ey/ex	Z	P>Z
UWI	0.900	1.280	0.201
AGE	-0.243	-0.190	0.851
EDU	0.267	0.700	0.487

Source: Estimated.

Table 6.35 SHI MP Rural BPL

Logistic regression   Number of obs =2,307
LR chi2(4) =3.18
Prob> chi2 =0.5281
Log likelihood = -1438.3189   Pseudo R2=0.0011

SHI	Coef.	z	P>z
RWI	0.120	1.500	0.132
SEX	0.040	0.280	0.776
AGE	-0.003	-0.770	0.439
EDU	-0.034	-0.640	0.521
cons	0.688	2.720	0.007

Source: Estimated.

Results for MP Rural BPL Uneducated

Results of rural BPL uneducated respondents for MP are presented in Tables 6.35–6.39 and Tables 6.35(a)–6.39(a) below. None of the four explanatory variables including income (RWI), sex, age and education are significant for SHI, RSBY or PHI (Tables 6.35–6.39), nor is a responsiveness depicted for

Table 6.35(a) SHI MP Rural BPL

Delta-method
Average marginal effects   Number of obs=2,307
Model VCE: OIM

SHI	ey/ex	Z	P>Z
RWI	0.057	1.530	0.126
SEX	0.014	0.280	0.776
AGE	-0.042	-0.770	0.442
EDU	-0.004	-0.620	0.538

Source: Estimated.

Table 6.36 RSBY MP Rural BPL

Logistic regression
Number of obs =2,307
LR chi2(4) =4.91
Prob> chi2 =0.2965
Log likelihood = -1324.9745   Pseudo R2 =0.0018

RSBY	Coef.	z	P>z
RWI	-0.161	-1.900	0.058
SEX	-0.116	-0.770	0.441
AGE	0.002	0.430	0.669
EDU	0.045	0.820	0.414
cons	-0.755	-2.810	0.005

Source: estimated.

Table 6.36(a) RSBY MP Rural BPL

Delta-method
Average marginal effects   Number of obs =2,307
Model VCE: OIM

RSBY	ey/ex	Z	P>Z
RWI	-0.182	-1.880	0.060
SEX	-0.096	-0.770	0.442
AGE	0.056	0.430	0.669
EDU	0.013	0.840	0.403

Source: Estimated

these variables for any of the schemes (Tables 6.35(a)–6.39(a)). Even in the case of only female respondents, similar results are noticeable for PHI (Table 6.39 and 6.39(a)). Thus, these results do not throw much light on the nature of choice in regard to health insurance schemes for BPL rural respondents.

Only Females

Results for above BPL and Educated Rural MP Respondents

The results of above BPL rural respondents are presented in Tables 6.40–6.44 and Tables 6.40(a)–6.44(a) below. These indicate that income is negatively influential in choices relating to SHI and RSBY (Tables 6.40 and 6.41,) but is

Table 6.37 CHI MP Rural BPL

Logistic regression   Number of obs =2,307
LR chi2(2) =1.36
Prob> chi2=0.5070
Log likelihood = -22.254153   Pseudo R2 =0.0296

CHI	Coef.	z	P>z
RWI	-0.618	-0.530	0.594
AGE	0.041	1.000	0.318
cons	-7.957	-2.680	0.007

Source: Estimated.

Table 6.37(a) CHI MP Rural BPL

Delta-method
Average marginal effects   Number of obs =2,307
Model VCE: OIM

CHI	ey/ex	Z	P>Z
RWI	-0.941	-0.530	0.594
AGE	2.030	1.000	0.317

Source: Estimated.

Table 6.38 PHI MP Rural BPL

Logistic regression   Number of obs =2,307
LR chi2(4) =2.74
Prob> chi2 =0.6030
Log likelihood = -57.532937   Pseudo R2 =0.0232

PHI	Coef.	z	P>z
RWI	0.168	0.290	0.773
SEX	-0.351	-0.330	0.745
AGE	0.005	0.210	0.836
EDU	-1.401	-1.300	0.192
cons	-5.379	-2.770	0.006

Source: Estimated.

Table 6.38(a) PHI MP Rural BPL

Delta-method
Average marginal effects   Number of obs =2,307
Model VCE: OIM

PHI	ey/ex	z	P>z
RWI	0.255	0.290	0.773
SEX	-0.392	-0.330	0.745
AGE	0.262	0.210	0.836
EDU	-0.551	-1.300	0.193

Source: Estimated.

Table 6.39 PHI Females Only MP Rural BPL

Logistic regression   Number of obs =280
LR chi2(1) =0.00
Prob> chi2 =0.9498
Log likelihood = -6.6310212   Pseudo R2 =0.0003

PHI F	Coef.	z	P>z
AGE	0.005	0.060	0.950
cons	-5.892	-1.370	0.170

Table 6.39(a) PHI Females Only MP Rural BPL

Delta-method
Average marginal effects   Number of obs =280
Model VCE: OIM

PHI F	ey/ex	Z	P>Z
AGE	0.257	0.060	0.950

Source: Estimated.

positive but insignificant in regard to CHI (Table 6.42) and positive and significant for PHI (Table 6.43). The scheme of RSBY is negatively responsive to income (Table 6.41(a)) whereas private health insurance is positively responsive to income (Table 6.43(a)). Unlike other schemes, a positive and significant influence of education is noted for choice of private health insurance (Table 6.43). However, unlike other results, the results for female respondents in above BPL rural MP do not show any significant variable in regard to private health insurance choices (Table 6.44 and 6.44(a)).

Table 6.40 SHI Above BPL MP

Logistic regression   Number of obs=2,215
LR chi2(4) =18.53
Prob> chi2 =0.0010
Log likelihood = -1392.6294   Pseudo R2 =0.0066

SHI	Coef.	z	P>z
RWI	-0.169	-2.930	0.003
SEX	-0.003	-0.010	0.991
AGE	-0.006	-1.790	0.073
EDU	-0.109	-2.110	0.035
cons	1.873	5.040	0.000

Source: Estimated.

Table 6.40(a) SHI Above BPL MP

Delta-method
Average marginal effects   Number of obs =2,215
Model VCE: OIM

SHI	ey/ex	Z	P>Z
RWI	-0.224	-2.870	0.004
SEX	-0.001	-0.010	0.991
AGE	-0.096	-1.760	0.078
EDU	-0.065	-2.040	0.041

Source: Estimated.

Table 6.41 RSBY Above BPL MP

Logistic regression
Number of obs =2,215
LR chi2(4) =24.19
Prob> chi2 =0.0001
Log likelihood = -1001.5695   Pseudo R2=0.0119

RSBY	Coef.	z	P>z
RWI	-0.345	-4.720	0.000
SEX	-0.287	-0.870	0.385
AGE	0.005	1.130	0.257
EDU	0.048	0.750	0.454
cons	-0.250	-0.520	0.603

Source: Estimated.

Table 6.41(a) RSBY Above BPL MP

Delta-method
Average marginal effects   Number of obs =2,215
Model VCE: OIM

RSBY	ey/ex	Z	P>Z
RWI	-1.144	-4.670	0.000
SEX	-0.247	-0.870	0.385
AGE	0.188	1.140	0.255
EDU	0.070	0.750	0.453

Source: Estimated.

Table 6.42 CHI Above BPL MP

Logistic regression   Number of obs =2,215
LR chi2(3) =2.64
Prob> chi2 =0.4503
Log likelihood = -78.435934   Pseudo R2 =0.0166

CHI	Coef.	z	P>z
RWI	0.116	0.330	0.741
AGE	0.032	1.570	0.117
EDU	0.057	0.190	0.849
cons	-7.224	-4.160	0.000

Source: Estimated.

Table 6.42(a) CHI Above BPL MP

Delta-method
Average marginal effects   Number of obs =2,215
Model VCE: OIM

CHI	ey/ex	Z	P>Z
RWI	0.457	0.330	0.741
AGE	1.425	1.570	0.117
EDU	0.101	0.190	0.849

Source: Estimated.

Table 6.43 PHI Above BPL MP

Logistic regression   Number of obs =2,215
LR chi2(4) =64.15
Prob> chi2 =0.0000
Log likelihood = -302.22955   Pseudo R2 =0.0959

PHI	Coef.	z	P>z
RWI	1.178	6.220	0.000
SEX	0.540	1.110	0.266
AGE	0.008	0.860	0.390
EDU	0.272	2.920	0.003
cons	-9.841	-9.040	0.000

Source: Estimated.

Table 6.43(a) PHI Above BPL MP

Delta-method
Average marginal effects   Number of obs=2,215
Model VCE: OIM

PHI	ey/ex	Z	P>Z
RWI	4.475	6.240	0.000
SEX	0.541	1.110	0.266
AGE	0.335	0.860	0.389
EDU	0.462	2.940	0.003

Source: Estimated.

Only Females

Table 6.44 PHI Above BPL Females MP

Logistic regression   Number of obs =85
LR chi2(3) =2.87
Prob> chi2 =0.4127
Log likelihood = -17.582868   Pseudo R2 =0.0754

PHI F	Coef.	z	P>z
RWI	1.092	1.450	0.148
AGE	-0.027	-0.650	0.517
EDU	0.018	0.040	0.969
cons	-6.360	-1.630	0.104

Source: Estimated.

Table 6.44(a) PHI Above BPL Females MP

Delta-method
Average marginal effects   Number of obs =85
Model VCE: OIM

PHI F	ey/ex	Z	P>Z
RWI	4.176	1.450	0.146
AGE	-1.159	-0.650	0.519
EDU	0.026	0.040	0.969

Source: Estimated.

Notes

1 Arrow (1963) also provided results for the optimal design of health insurance. He showed that if insurance is not actuarially fair (which it never truly is) and if utility is not state dependent, the optimal health insurance contract was full insurance above a deductible. Later, Arrow (1974) showed that with health state dependent utility the optimal deductible fluctuates depending on how marginal utility varies with health status. (see for instance, Gerfin, 2019).

2 Over the years in the literature on health insurance focus has been on either only on demand side (for instance Pauly, 1968); Zeckhauser, 1970 and other researchers) or supply side (like McGuire, 2000); or both like Chandra, Cutler, and Song, 2012; . Arokiasamy Perianayagam and Srinivas Goli, 2013.

    In the Indian context, see, for instance, Berman, 1998; Ellis *et al.*, 2000; Kutzin, 2001; Mahal, 2002; Ahuja, 2004; Wagstaff et al., 2009.

3 See, for instance, Purohit Brijesh C. (2013), Demand for Healthcare in India, Healthcare in Low-resource Settings 2013; 1:e7].

4 International Institute of Population Sciences, *National Family Health Survey, 2015-16*, Government of India.

Chapter 7

Conclusions and Policy Imperatives

India has achieved important milestones due to sustained, planned efforts. Despite the achievements with the prevailing national and state health policies and the systematic five-year plan health sector priorities, there are numerous disconcerting features and newly emerging issues in the health care sector in India. While India's total population is more than 16 per cent of the total global population, it accounts for a large share of (nearly one-fifth) of the global diseases. In fact, of the latter, a large incidence and prevalence of diseases in India, such as diarrhoeal diseases, TB, respiratory and parasitic infections, maternal conditions, nutritional deficiencies, diabetes, venereal diseases and HIV/AIDS cases, comprise a considerable chunk of diseases. As a result, India needs to have a health system which can cater to our vast population and address this burden of diseases efficiently and effectively.

However, by contrast, the overall state financing of the health care sector in India, as noted earlier, has been inadequate. There is also an unsatisfactory distribution of infrastructure and resources in the health care sector. This has led to undesirable outcomes, which is prominently noted in widespread disparity in health care services in rural and urban areas, poor and rich states and a notable neglect of some of the emerging health needs of the society.

Further, despite a systematic planned effort, there is an unsatisfactory situation depicted in regard to the public sector, particularly in health care. This is owing to the developed three-tier health system with its large network of primary health centres, district hospitals and advanced medical research and teaching, as well as specialised hospitals, but which remains considerably constrained by lack of medicines, material and manpower. Even the low public investment is largely spent (nearly 70 per cent) in recurring expenditure (including wages and salaries) and a very small amount is spent on medicines and drugs for patients' care. Estimates indicate a real per capita health care expenditure as Rs. 120 only. In terms of international comparison, in 2016, for instance, India's per capita expenditure (US$62) has been much lower than China (US$398), Sri Lanka (US$153) and Bhutan (US$91).

Therefore, a major role seems to have been assigned inadvertently to the private sector. Moreover, with currently prevailing patterns, the private

DOI: 10.4324/9781032615660-7

health care sector can be considered as more inequitable and less regulated. The situation in regard to the social security (or insurance through budgetary expenditure including health) and private insurance in health is also not satisfactory, which is evident from their overall contribution to social security/ health insurance in the year 2016 to the tune of 6 per cent and 4 per cent, respectively. Yet as per NFHS 4 survey (2016), cumulatively, all public sector facilities/providers catered to nearly 53 per cent of overall health care utilisation across India. Within the public sector, a major share of the provision of health care facilities has been through three sources; government/municipal hospitals (22.33 per cent), CHC (14 per cent) and PHCs (11 per cent) (see Chapter 2). Against this, within a 47 per cent share of utilisation by the private providers in all India scenarios, the major shares were from private doctors (27 per cent) and private hospitals (14 per cent).

Despite higher utilisation of public health care facilities, there is inadequate medical manpower and beds in public hospitals. This was noted by a high-level expert group on Universal Health Coverage at Erstwhile Planning Commission, and it was noted that this situation would mean it would take at least 17 years to reach World Health Organization's norm of one doctor per 1000 people. At present, as per a World Health Organization report 2017) on the Health Workforce in India, on average, there are 64.9 physicians per one lakh people in the country.

In the earlier chapters, we have discussed both aspects, namely the health care system and health insurance system in the country in greater detail in order to look into possible strategies that could help the people's health care needs through a better mix of the roles of public and private sectors. Thus, we provide some possible ways by which both the health care and health insurance sectors could cater better in times to come that may help us to achieve SDG targets and move towards universal health insurance coverage.

It is worth recalling that in the country there are as many as 22 health insurance schemes that are also functioning as public sector government financed schemes. However, most of the central and state government sponsored schemes do not have provisions for taking care of outpatient expenditure. This puts many people utilising such schemes into financial difficulties due to large out of pocket expenses on OPD care. Thus, it is important that governments look into the possibility of incorporating this component in the state sponsored scheme. This could be done by adjusting the basic fees and a better negotiation with the public or private insurer. Another important thing is to take care of the current situation of low efficiency of health insurance, which is caused by health insurance being an unprofitable business for insurance companies, owing to the high claims ratio which has exceeded 100 per cent in many cases for both public and private insurers. In order to overcome this, there should be an increased role of public-private partnerships in insurance, in terms of increasing coverage and thus increasing volume of business. Since the increase in the number of insured people will not result in adverse selection and moral hazard problems, there is a likelihood that, in due course, utilisation levels of health care facilities under the state sponsored schemes will stabilise to provide an incentive to insurers, through a reduced claim ratio. This suggestion takes into account the fact that: (a) the claims ratio is only 76 per cent in individual insurance of health, which is lower than group insurance under state sponsored schemes, and (b) despite a trend of growing health insurance business, in group insurance segments and overall number of persons covered are the highest in government sponsored schemes (77 per cent). By contrast, the group and individual insurance coverage in numbers is only 16 and 7 per cent, respectively. This suggestion may also help to make public sector insurance companies more financially self-sufficient, and it may also provide private insurance companies the opportunity to increase their business in health insurance, which currently comprises a very low proportion of their overall business. Lastly, it is also worth mentioning that until we are sure of the depth and reach of national health insurance schemes like RSBY and proposed Ayusman Bharat, we should retain the uniqueness of prevailing state sponsored schemes in different states, such that political incentive and socio-economic milieu of state specific nature are retained and sustained even with a universal health insurance.

Bibliography

Ahuja, R. (2004). "Health insurance for the poor." *Economic and Political Weekly* 34(28): 3171–3178.

Arrow, K. J. (1963). "Uncertainty and the welfare economics of medical care." *American Economic Review* 53: 941–973.

Arrow, K. J. (1968). "The economics of moral hazard: Further comment." *American Economic Review* 58: 537–539.

Arrow, K. J. (1974). "Optimal insurance and generalized deductibles." *Scandinavian Actuarial Journal* (1): 1–42.

Berman, P. (1998). "Rethinking health care systems: Private health care provision in India." *World Development* 26(8): 1463–1479.

Chandra, A., D. Cutler, and Z. Song (2012). "Who ordered that? The economics of treatment choices in medical care." *Handbook of Health Economics* 2: 397–432. Amsterdam: Elsevier.

Ellis, R., M. Alam, and I. Gupta (2000). "Health Insurance in India: Prognosis & prospectus." *Economic & Political Weekly* 22: 207–216.

Gerfin, Michael (2019). *Health Insurance and the Demand for Healthcare*; Online Publication Date: March. DOI: 10.1093/acrefore/9780190625979.013.257

Kutzin, J. (2001). "A descriptive framework for country level analysis of health care financing arrangements." *Health Policy* 56: 171–204.

Mahal, A. (2002). "Assessing private health insurance in India: Political impact and regulatory issue." *Economic and Political Weekly* 5: 59–71.

McGuire, T. G. (2000). "Physician agency." In edited by A. J. Culyer and J. P. Newhouse *Handbook of Health Economics* (Vol. 1). Amsterdam: Elsevier, pp. 461–536.

Pauly, M. V. (1968). "The economics of moral hazard: Comment." *American Economic Review* 58: 531–537.

Perianayagam, Arokiasamy and Srinivas Goli (2013). "Health insurance and health care in India: A supply-demand perspective." International Institute for Population Sciences (IIPS), Giri Institute of Development Studies (GIDS), 31 October MPRA Paper No. 51103, posted 1 November 2013 09:52 UTC; Online at https://mpra.ub.uni-muenchen.de/51103/.

Wagstaff, A., M. Lindelow, G. Junc, X. Ling, and Q. Juncheng (2009). "Extending health insurance to the rural population: An impact evaluation of China's new cooperative 102 medical schemes." *Journal of Health Economics* 28: 1–9.

Zeckhauser, R. (1970). "Medical insurance: A case study of the tradeoff between risk spreading and appropriate incentives." *Journal of Economic Theory* 2: 10–26.

Chapter 8

Role of Health Insurance in Post-pandemic Time

Pre-COVID, the number of people who purchased comprehensive insurance plans in India was approximately 32 per cent, whereas now, after being hit by one of the biggest pandemics in the history, this has shot up to 55 per cent.

The COVID-19 pandemic has resulted in an increased health insurance need worldwide. After SARS in 2002 and MERS in 2012, which limited their havoc to specific regions, the coronavirus has infected more than 147 million people and claimed more than three million lives. This health crisis has resulted in high inflation, especially medical inflation, and unemployment in the country.

COVID-19 has huge treatment costs, which has affected the finances and well-being of different sections of society, especially the poor and the middle-class. Thus, more and more people are considering health insurance coverage after such a pandemic as essential for survival. In India, where insurance penetration is below 4 per cent, it becomes a priority, among other essential things. The result is an increase in comprehensive health insurance to 55 per cent in contrast to earlier comparable figures of 32 per cent.

The changes that occurred in India have also been considerable due to the clause of the Insurance Regulatory and Development Authority of India (IRDAI) in July 2020, that all health insurance providers are now mandated to provide coverage for COVID-19 treatment under their regular health insurance plan. This is termed as Corona Kavach Plan and Corona Rakshak Plan. These two plans were specially designed to help policyholders meet the healthcare cost incurred due to the coronavirus disease. The regulator had also earlier in the year launched a Standard Health Insurance Product (SHIP) by the name Arogya Sanjeevani Policy to help people enjoy standard and comprehensive health insurance coverage. Moreover the current Prime Minister's Jan Arogya Yojana (PMJAY) has benefitted some of the middle and lower income segments in some of the States. Thus, overall, an increased awareness has been created regarding the importance of health and health insurance plans. It has made us come to terms with how crucial it is to remain financially shielded as emergencies, especially medical emergencies, come

DOI: 10.4324/9781032615660-8

without a warning sign and can result in financial strain along with emotional grief (Agarwal, 2021).

> In the Indian context, it would be useful if a universal program could be conceived that covers everyone from birth to death. Like India, some other countries also found it more feasible to achieve universal coverage through compulsory health insurance administered by insurance companies under close regulation and supervision by the government. The intent and effect of such programs is similar to that achieved by tax supported public insurance.
>
> Now looking back in the recent past, it could be said that the pre-pandemic health care system was inefficient. When insurance is paying the costs of medical services, patients want any care that offers some expected benefit, regardless of cost
>
> (Victor, 2020)

COVID-19 has led all countries to renew commitment to improve health as a central component of the sustainable development goals (SDGs) agenda. The concept of universal health coverage requires health system strengthening around people, institutions and resources to build a resilient health system to provide a timely response to emergencies through detection and prevention, while maintaining peace and protecting the economy. Those countries with effective universal health coverage, such as South Korea and Singapore, have performed better during the COVID-19 pandemic. Even the health systems of some of the world's wealthiest nations affected by the pandemic pointed to inadequate healthcare facilities and lack of resources such as shortages of hospital beds, medicines, ventilators and healthcare workforce.

Notably the countries most affected by the pandemic (like the United States) are the ones that have done little in the past to strengthen their health system through appropriate investment in universal health coverage. As indicated by Amirhossein et al. (2020), on the other hand, Iran is facing a unique paradox. Though it has transformed its health system to achieve universal health coverage for more than 90 per cent (of its 83 million population) and despite its well-established primary healthcare network and increased access to quality care and comprehensive programmes for prevention and control of non-communicable diseases, it is among the top Asian nations affected by COVID-19. This is partly due not only to shortcomings in integrating emergency response into primary health care, but also to US sanctions hampering investment in and access to medicines and essential equipment.

In the USA, for instance, in 2022, more than 75 million cases of COVID-19 were tracked. Health insurers were responsible for covering certain forms of COVID-19 testing.

Due to the pandemic shutdowns of restaurants, office buildings, gyms, sports and entertainment venues and other businesses occurred. Consequently, unemployment in the U.S. rose sharply from 3.5 per cent in January 2020 to 14.7 per cent in April, and more than 20 million people lost their jobs in April alone.

Because employment is the primary source of health insurance coverage for Americans, the record-setting jobs losses took an even greater toll. Even though many unemployed people gained coverage through Medicaid and Marketplace plans, nearly 3 million people still lost health insurance during the spring and summer of 2020.

To overcome this lack of health insurance, the government had taken steps to provide a safety net and combat the rapid decline of employer-based coverage rates. Also, a legislation called The Families First Coronavirus Response Act prohibited states from terminating Medicaid coverage during the pandemic, and the Affordable Care Act had expanded Medicaid coverage to all low-income adults in many states. However, the number of people who lost health insurance coverage due to unemployment was higher in states that had not expanded Medicaid.

Another Act, the No Surprises Act, which took effect January 1, 2022, and protected insured patients from receiving unexpected bills for healthcare they had received from out-of-network hospitals, doctors or providers they did not select. As an example, research shows roughly one in five emergency room visits result in surprise bills due to patients inadvertently receiving out-of-network care.

The No Surprises Act also includes the following provisions:

- It required private health plans to cover out-of-network claims and apply in network cost sharing. The law applies to both job-based and non-group plans.
- It prohibited doctors, hospitals and other covered providers from billing patients more than the in-network cost sharing amount for surprise medical bills.

Providers were obligated to make policyholders aware of those protections, and both providers and health plans were responsible for identifying bills that are protected under the Act.

Behavioural shifts also increased urgent care centres visits by 58 per cent. Out of this increase, first-time visitors accounted for nearly half of the 28 million patients who used urgent care. This suggests that urgent care centres also offer patients greater convenience. Overall, urgent care providers have higher rates of technology adoption compared to the primary care sector. The growing reliance on urgent care also helps reduce emergency room visits, which helps conserve hospital resources and results in lower costs for carriers and patients alike (BDO, 2023).

Insurers should assess the impact in five areas in the post-pandemic era:

1. To offer workers more flexibility in coverage options, organisations are increasingly turning to health reimbursement arrangements (HRAs) and self-insurance options.
2. Insurance should be used as an incentive, such that in future provision of charging unvaccinated employees more for health insurance to cover the increased risk of hospitalisation with a condition caused by any pandemic.
3. Increasing coverage of telehealth services. For instance, in the USA, Johns Hopkins researchers found a more than 50-fold increase in telehealth use among privately insured people of working age and one market research firm even forecasted a sevenfold growth in the telehealth market by 2025.
4. Insurers should take into consideration the need for care for long COVID cases which means COVID-19 survivors who develop new symptoms and receive new diagnoses up to six months after their initial bout with the virus. Those who've received such diagnoses are thought to be suffering from "long COVID." These include symptoms like fatigue, brain fog and cardiac complications. Thus, the definition of "medical necessity" may need reconsideration (BDO, 2023).
5. Growing emphasis on mental health to include the phenomenon of isolation, fears of contracting the virus and economic uncertainty creating a growing mental health crisis and therefore, a suitable provision in insurance coverage for mental health services.

As a UN policy brief of 2020 indicates, the focus of countries should be on following areas:

(a) Invest in core health systems functions that are fundamental to protecting and promoting health and well-being, known as "common goods for health". Governments need to expand their investments in common goods for health so that the world does not face this situation again when outbreaks occur. Having these functions in place is integral to the commitments all Member States made in the International Health Regulations, as well as the Political Declaration on Universal Health Coverage in 2019. These include policy coordination, surveillance, communication, regulation for quality products, fiscal instruments and subsidies to public health programmes. (b) Suspend user fees for COVID-19 and other essential health care. The reduction of financial barriers to service use is an important measure for countries to move towards universal health coverage. Ideally, patients do not have to worry about paying user fees at the point of care because, particularly at this time, financial considerations should not enter an individual's calculus as to whether and where to seek care. Public and contracted private providers could be compensated by advanced provider payments where feasible during the COVID-19 pandemic.

(UN, 2020)

Additionally, considering the example of four countries (Savedoff, 2004) including Britain, Malaysia, Brazil and Sweden, representing a range of experiences with Tax-Based Systems for universal health insurance, some relevant direction for our country can be thought of for adopting universal health insurance coverage. Among these, in Britain, Malaysia and Brazil, financing is based on national revenues, while Sweden's public health services rely largely on local taxes. Britain and Malaysia have strong national management of the health services, while Sweden and Brazil have decentralised models with local management of services. Britain, Sweden and Malaysia have effectively reached their goal of universal access, while Brazil is as yet unsuccessful in this regard. In each case, establishing the system required a political movement focused on universalising access to health care. Apart from Malaysia, each country established its Tax-Based System on a foundation that had been laid by the growth of social insurance plans. Thus, the basic infrastructure for health care services and payment mechanisms was already in place. The budget for government-financed health care services is determined through political processes – forcing health care to compete with a variety of other government services for funds. Sweden's government health care services are already highly decentralised; but Britain, Brazil and, to a lesser extent, Malaysia are all moving in that direction. In fact, reforms in Brazil, Britain and Sweden already presumed that health services should be largely financed with government revenues. The scope and quality of services differs across these countries, with reasonably good performance in Britain, Sweden and Malaysia. Along with rising incomes and expectations, the private sector has expanded in each of these countries – the least in Sweden. The outcomes are based on the interplay of political parties and employers. Thus, these countries have achieved many of the positive goals set by public policy – universal access, rising health status and moderate costs. However, moving towards Tax-Based Systems also has the problems of health service provision, which have been debated over the years for other public merit goods provision. It also resonates the oft familiar discussions like consumption versus income taxes, national versus local, and earmarked versus general. In part, it results from expectations for faster and more responsive health services. In India, to some, it has been performed by central or state finance commissions. These commissions have helped in changing allocation formulas and decentralising responsibilities.

References

Agrawal, Ankit (2021). "The ever growing need for health insurance post pandemic." *Financial Express*, June 7.

Amirhossein, Takian, Mohsen Aarabi, and Hajar Haghighi. (2020). "The role of universal health coverage in overcoming the Covid-19 pandemic." *BMJ.com*, April 20.

BDO (2023). USA LLP, a Delaware limited partnership; online website.

Savedoff, William (2004). Tax-based financing for health systems: Options and experiences. Discussion paper, No. 4 – 2004, Department "Health System Financing, Expenditure and Resource Allocation" (FER) Cluster "Evidence and Information for Policy" (EIP World Health Organisation), Geneva, 2004.

United Nations (2020). Covid 19 and Universal Health Coverage: Policy Brief, October 20, United Nations, USA.

Victor, Fuchs R. (2020). "Health care policy after the COVID-19 pandemic." *JAMA* 324(3). Published Online: June 12, 2020. doi:10.1001/jama.2020.10777.

Index

Page numbers in **bold** denote tables, those in *italic* denote figures.

65th World Health Assembly (WHA) (2013) 22

Above All India Average States (AAIAS) 14–17, *20–22*, **24**, 27, **29**, *30*, *34–36*, **46–47**, 48–50, **58**, 60, **63**
Ahlin, Tanja 109
Ahmad, Nabi 76
Alma Ata declaration (1978) 5
Amirhossein, Takian 194
Arogya Karnataka (Karnataka Arogya Bhagya) 115
AYUSH 15–16, **28–29**, *30*, **31**, *34*, **41–48**, **51**, 67–68, **70**, **91**, 102–103
Ayushman Bharat (MODI Care) 3, 107–109, 117–121, 127

Below All India Average States (BAIAS) 14–17, *20–22*, **25**, 27, **29**, *30*, *34–36*, **43–45**, 47–48, *50*, **57**, 60, **63**
below poverty line (BPL) 63, 80–83, 89, **101**, 108, 111–116, **125–126**, 152–153, **154**, 157–159, 163, **164**, 167, **168–175**, 176–180, **181–188**
benefits 8, 75–77, 79, **88**, 89, **93–100**, 111, 113–114, 116, 121, 128, **136–138**, 149, **150**, 152
Bhore Committee 1, 8
budgetary expenditure 9, 11, 15, 107, 113, 190

central government health insurance scheme (CGHS) **28**, 53, 63, 64, **66**, 67–69 **70–72**, *73*, 74, **90–92**, 110, 116, **126**, 127, 157

Central Services Medical Attendance (CSMA) 63
Chauhan, Tarun 108
Choudhury, Mita 111
community health centres (CHCs) 1, 17, **18–19**, 21, **33**, **41–48**, 49–50, 190
community health financing 134, 139, 152
COVID-19 193–194, 196–197

Dhingra, Reeta 135
disability adjusted life years (DALY) Index 7

Employees' State Insurance Act (1948) 75
Employees State Insurance Scheme (ESIS) 53, 63–64, **66**, 75–76, **77–79**, **93**, **95**, **97–100**, **102–103**, **126**, 127, 157
Ex-Serviceman Contributory Health Scheme 64, **66**, **126**

family planning 5, 7, **15**, **53**, **61**
Five Year Plans 5–6, 8, **51**, 189; First (1951–1956) 5–6, **51**; Second (1956–1961) 5, **51**; Third (1961–1966) 5, **51**; Fourth (1969–1974) 5, **51**; Fifth (1974–1979) 5, **51**; Sixth (1980–1984) 5, **51**; Seventh (1985–1990) 6, **51**; Eighth (1992–1997) 6, **51**; Ninth (1997–2002) 2, 6, **51**; Tenth (2002–2007) 6, **51**, 69; Eleventh (2007–2012) 6, **51**; Twelfth (2012–2017) 6, **51**
Forgia, Gerard La 110

Garg Charu, C. 110
Government of India (GOI) 2, 6, 10, 81–82, 111
Government Sponsored Health Insurance Scheme (GSHISs) 107, 109–110

Health and Wellness centres 118
health care 1–2, 9, 32, 46, 111, 118, 128, 189–190, 197; access to 80, 197; ambulatory 53; costs 2; deficiencies 2; delivery 1–2; demand for 119, 156; essential 196; expenditure 8, 12, *16–17*, **62**, 119, 189; facilities 6, 9, 12, *18*, 45, 48, 60, 69, 190–191; financing of 9, 134; functions 52; government funded 117, 197; industry 2; investments in 81; needs 190; oral 111–112; practitioners **15**; pre-pandemic 194; primary 1, 32, 194; private 2, 9, 46, 83; providers 1, **15, 53**, 63, 89; public 190; quality of 8, 74, 110; secondary 1, 153; sector 2, 6, 8, 189–190; services 2, 12, **52**, 63, 74, 83, 87, 115, 189, 197; tertiary 1; treatment 116; universal 2, 109, 118; utilisation 2, 109, 118, 134, 190; *see also* mental health
Health for All 5, 115
health insurance: schemes 2, 64, *65*, **66**, 81, 85, 107–117, 120–121, **125**, 127–128, 130, 134–135, **136**, 139, 152, 167, 176, 182, 190–191; systems 190
Health Policy of India (1983, 2002, 2017) 1
Highest Education Level (HEL) 158, **159–175**
human resources 7, 21, 26, 33

ICMR/ICSSR Report 5
immunisation 7, **52**, 74, **103**
Insurance Regulatory and Development Authority (IRDA) 2, 82, 130–131, 193
investment 5–6, 8, 29, **51**, 81, 119, 189, 194, 196

Jain, Kalpana 89, 111
Jose, Mathew 77
Jyotiba Phule Jan Arogya Yojana, Maharashtra (MJPJAY) **66**, 115

Kumari, Aparajita 74

maternal and child health (MCH) services 5, 67
mental disability 18
mental health 6, 17–18, 21–22, 26–27, 31–33, 39, 41–43, 196; care 19, 22, 27; crisis 196; disorders 38; financing 39; hospitals **15, 53**; interventions 21; issues 20; needs 29, 33; Policy 17, 22, 32; problems 18, 22, 26–27, 29, 32; programme 19–20, 30–31, 39; promotion of 21, 26, 32–33; services 21–22, 33, 196; situation 17; specialists 39; status 34
mental illness 18–19, 30–32, 34; orphaned persons with (OPMI) 27; prevalence **36**, 41; prevention of 33; severity of 18, 34; untreated 19
MERS (2012) 193
Millennium Development Goals (MDGs) 60
Ministry of Health and Family Welfare 10, **103**, 113
MODI Care *see* Ayushman Bharat
mortality 108; high 6; neo-natal 7; premature 7
mortality rates **61–62**; infant (IMR) 6–7, 9; maternal (MMR) 6–7, **61**; road traffic **61**; suicide **61**

Nagaraju, Y. 109
Nandi, S. 112
National Family Health Survey 2015–2016 (NFHS-4) 2, **42**, 45, 48, *49*, 113, 156–157, 176, 190
National Food Security Scheme (NFSS) 115
National Health accounts (NHA) 10, **12**, **15**, **52**, 57, 63–64, **66**
National Health Information Network 8
National Health Policy 5–9, 16, 113, 118–120
National Institute of Mental Health and Neurosciences (NIMHANS) 33, 41–42
National Mental Health Policy 17, 22
National Mental Health Programme 19, 39
National Mental Health Survey 33
No Surprises Act (2022) 195

out-of-pocket (OOP) expenses 86–87,
108, 134

Panda, Pradeep 135
Post 2015 Development Agenda 60
primary health centres (PHCs) 1, 4, 5, 8,
17, **18–19**, *20*, **33**, **41–48**, 49–51, **53**,
152–153, 189–190
Privately Purchased Health Insurance
Plan (PHI) 157–158, 176–177,
178–181, 182, **183–184**, **187–188**
Public Health Resource Network 117
public-private partnership (PPP) 2, 69,
102–103, 108, 114, 127, 190

Quantitative Goals and Objectives 7

Rajasekhar, D. 110
Ranson, M. Kent 135
Rashtriya Swasthya Bima Yojana
(RSBY) **66**, 80, **82**, **84–86**
Rathi, A. 109
rehabilitation 18, 30, 109–110, **136**,
138; allowance 75; physical **94**;
vocational 75
Rural Wealth Index (RWI) 158–159,
160–167, **181–188**

SARS (2002) 193
Sarwal, Rakesh 110
Sharma, A. N. 111
Shekhar, Vrishali 109–110
social security 11, 77, 190;
expenditure **12**; health insurance
schemes 81, 127

socio-economic Caste Census (SECC)
117, 120
Sood, Neeraj 108
sub-centres (SCs) **1**, **4**, **18**, *20*, 45, **53**
substance use **14**, **39–140**, 42, 44
Sustainable Development Agenda 60
Sustainable Development Goals (SDGs)
2–3, 60, **61–62**, 190, 194

Thomas, K. T. 109
three-tier system 1
total health expenditure (THE) 10, **12**,
57–58, 60, **62**

United Nations General Assembly 60
universal health; care 2, 109, 118;
coverage (UHC) 110
Universal Health Insurance Scheme
(UHIS) 111, 130
US Affordable Care Act 121

Vajpayee Arogyashree scheme 108
Vellakkal, S. S. 72
Venkitasubramanian, Akshay 108

water supply and sanitation 2
wealth index value 157
well-being 17, 193, 196; mental 18;
social 18
World Bank 81, 119
World Health Organization (WHO) 1,
18, 119, 124, 190

For Product Safety Concerns and Information please contact our EU
representative GPSR@taylorandfrancis.com
Taylor & Francis Verlag GmbH, Kaufingerstraße 24, 80331 München, Germany

* 9 7 8 1 0 3 2 6 1 5 6 5 3 *